PROGRESS IN CLINICAL PHARMACY: V

Concept and practice of therapeutic teams

This book reports the proceedings of the eleventh European symposium on clinical pharmacy which was held in Brussels in October 1982. The theme of the symposium was the concept of the therapeutic team and the relative contributions and responsibilities of pharmacists, nurses and physicians to the planning and implementation of drug treatment regimens.

The first section of the volume provides an introduction to the concept of the therapeutic team and reflects the views of a pharmacist, of an academic, of a nurse, of a physician and of a clinical pharmacologist. The later sections cover the practice of the therapeutic team in parenteral nutrition, oncology, dermatology, epilepsy, internal medicine, nuclear medicine and drug selection. In addition, a series of exciting prospects in the practice of the teams were developed in the free communications and poster sessions of the symposium and these are included in the volume, which therefore provides a very important document in clinical pharmacy.

Not only does this book review current achievements and experiences in clinical pharmacy, but it also provides stimulating discussions that look towards the exciting future of clinical pharmacy development in Europe.

PROGRESS IN CLINICAL PHARMACY: V

Concept and Practice of Therapeutic Teams

Proceedings of the 11th European Symposium
on Clinical Pharmacy, Brussels 1982

Edited by

H. DE CLERCQ
Director of Pharmacy Services, Academic Ziekenhuis
Vrije Universiteit Brussels

J. W. POSTON
Lecturer Clinical and Social Pharmacy, Welsh School of Pharmacy,
UWIST, Cardiff

JOAQUIN BONAL
President, European Society of Clinical Pharmacy
Director of Pharmacy Services
Hospital Sta. Creu i Sant Pau, Barcelona

CAMBRIDGE UNIVERSITY PRESS
Cambridge
London   New York   New Rochelle
Melbourne   Sydney

CAMBRIDGE UNIVERSITY PRESS
Cambridge, New York, Melbourne, Madrid, Cape Town,
Singapore, São Paulo, Delhi, Tokyo, Mexico City

Cambridge University Press
The Edinburgh Building, Cambridge CB2 8RU, UK

Published in the United States of America by Cambridge University Press, New York

www.cambridge.org
Information on this title: www.cambridge.org/9780521279178

© Cambridge University Press 1983

First published 1983
First paperback edition 2011

A catalogue record for this publication is available from the British Library

Library of Congress Catalogue Card Number: 83–1958

ISBN 978-0-521-25595-0 Hardback
ISBN 978-0-521-27917-8 Paperback

CONTENTS

Contents

PREFACE

The 11th European Symposium on Clinical Pharmacy was held in Brussels, Belgium during 20–22 October 1982. The pre-congress and the symposium were attended by 254 scientists from 17 countries – USA, Norway, Sweden, Finland, Denmark, Iceland, Switzerland, Germany, Austria, Spain, Portugal, Italy, France, United Kingdom, Zimbabwe, the Netherlands and Belgium – all of whom actively participated in the meetings, poster sessions, learning resource center and scientific exhibition.

The general committee consisted of J. Bonal (Spain, President), G. Aulagner (France), H. Turakka (Finland), D. Schaaf (Germany), P. Amacker (Switzerland), B. Davidson (Sweden), H. De Clercq (Belgium), S. Ellis (United Kingdom), E. van der Kleijn (the Netherlands) and G. Ostino (Italy). The local scientific organisation for the meeting was carried out by H. De Clercq (Chairman), M. Delanghe (Secretary), P. Bruyneel (Treasurer), G. Algoet, A. Mathieu, and members of the staff at Brussels (AZ-VUB) and Leuven (AZ St Raphaël) University Hospitals, together with J. Van Nuwenborg and his colleagues at the AZ-St Jan Hospital Brugge.

The theme of the symposium was the concept of the therapeutic team and the relative contribution and responsibilities of pharmacists, nurses and physicians to the planning and implementation of drug treatment regimens. The scientific discussions were divided into eight main sections with 36 invited and 30 contributed papers. The meeting started with a detailed visit of the clinical pharmacy department of the AZ-St Jan Hospital in Brugge. This provided an opportunity to share achievements and experiences in the development of haemodialysis.

The first session of the symposium provided an introduction to the concept of the therapeutic team, and reflected the views of a pharmacist, of an academic, of a nurse, of a physician and of a clinical pharmacologist. Seven sessions covered the practice of the therapeutic team in parenteral nutrition, oncology, dermatology, epilepsy, internal medicine, nuclear medicine and drug selection. In addition, a series of exciting prospects in the practice of the teams were developed in the free communication and poster sessions.

This book contains all the lectures presented at the meeting. Therefore, it provides a very important document in clinical pharmacy; not only reviewing current achievements and experiences in clinical pharmacy services, but also providing stimulating discussions that look towards the exciting future of clinical pharmacy development in Europe.

I would like to express my thanks to all members of the organising committee for their assistance in organising the meeting, to Mady Gillet and the members of her staff for carrying out the local organisation, to the authors for promptly producing their manuscripts for this volume, and my secretary, Myriam Verhasselt, for her invaluable assistance.

Henri L. O. De Clercq

Academisch Ziekenhuis,
Vrije Universiteit Brussel
December 1982

INTRODUCTORY REMARKS

Concept and practice of the therapeutic team.

H. De Clerq, J.W. Poston.

Team membership and the implying interprofessional relations
are simple yet important concepts that many professionals have failed to
develop and find difficult to systematically incorporate into their daily
practice. As opposed to our great grandfathers 100 years ago, contemporary
man generally does not have to battle the physical environment; modern
man is more likely to be involved with other people than with physical
objects. Indeed, the degree to which we succeed in life and in our
profession is largely determined by how well we are able to understand,
predict and cope with other people's demands and expectations.

Mass media such as radio, television, newspapers and
contemporary educational systems all emphasise the growing role of
behavioural sciences in modern society. Even our own professional
journals regularly feature articles on the psychosocial forces modern
pharmacists need to understand to get more closely involved in patient
care, and to develop good interprofessional relations with other
disciplines. (e.g. Hoop (1979), Provost (1980), Kilwein (1981,1982),
Dolinsky (1982)).

At this point, and before discussing the principles of teams
and the activities that could develop interprofessional relationships in
hospitals, it is first necessary to have a definition of the team.

A team is an interdisciplinary group of individuals working
together in order to study a distinct subject.

Since the orientation of today's symposium is a clinical one,
we can translate this definition as follows:

A therapeutic team is an interdisciplinary group of qualified
individuals, engaged in a collaborative system of providing health care.

The care is both direct, in the form of planning and

implementation of drug regimens for particular patients, and indirect in
the form of policy and procedure development to monitor therapeutic
activity.

One question raised, is for what reason did team approach
develop in the delivery of health care? The major reason is obvious:
the treatment of diseases is not a matter of isolated technical intervention, but depends on a large variety of disciplines. As a result of
this multi-professional approach, fragmentation occurs, the patient's
entity gradually fades away, and the total patient has to make room for
a clustering of disease processes, drugs and all sorts of bits and pieces
that vary with the perspectives of the practitioners involved.

Recent attempts such as an integrated approach to medicine,
patient-orientated pharmacy or patient-centred nursing care may have
succeeded in various degrees to humanise the health care system and to
treat human beings instead of just diseases – they did as such not solve
all of the practitioner's problems.

A second reason why team approach developed in the delivery
of health care, is the ever increasing specialisation of our professions
and the resulting fragmentary approach each discipline has taken in the
provision of health care.

Let's take an example from pharmacy: with more of the
hospital pharmacists participating in clinically orientated programs, the
tasks of the pharmacists – especially in large university research
orientated hospitals – become increasingly specialised. As a result, we
can see now, within the same hospital, a pharmacist in charge of the I.V.
admixture programme, another one responsible for the drug information
centre, yet other pharmacists in charge of purchasing, manufacturing,
quality control, unit dose distribution, radiopharmaceuticals, TPN,
satellite pharmacies on the nursing units, patient interviews for
accurate drug history, maintaining patient profiles, counselling patients
on drug compliance and the proper use of drugs etc.

This example, taken from the recent evolution of hospital
pharmacy, can of course mutatis mutandi equally apply to the advancing
degree of specialisation that can be found in any other health care
discipline.

As a result, the practitioner often grows over specialised in his own professional field, that within his own hospital he will hardly find any other expert he can talk with. Interacting communication becomes a problem then, and will eventually only be provided by either a horizontal flow process, i.e. within the specialisation area with other experts during symposia or congress meetings, or else by a vertical communication flow process i.e. a communication through all inter-dependant subsystems of the hospital.

At this point, team approach is the most efficient and effective structure to support this communication flow, thus fostering the development of what is called "interprofessional relations".

Multiprofessional team-work requires a few essential principles. One is that all of the members of the team are equal in the sense that each member is dependent on the activity and presence of the other members, and further, that the loss of one member (or activity) results in a lessening of the quality of services provided by the whole. As another principle, the team <u>dynamic</u> : the team composition changes as a function of the specific type of care that is to be provided.

This "team" then communicates and functions on two levels:

(1) through a formalised network of structures that exchange information consistently (e.g. departmental newsletters, medical rounds, committees etc.), and

(2) through an informal network without set form or consistency of exchange (e.g. coffee breaks, telephone conversations, hallway discussions etc.).

The department of pharmacy traditionally has directed its formal communications to members of the medical staff, reserved the informal patterns for nursing staff, and then often giving only perfunctory greetings to the remaining professional staff members.

These communication patterns tend to be ineffective for promoting interprofessional relationships and better patient care. This is however not the only problem.

Traditionally the medical and nursing professions have been defined as the team, and therefore must be presented with overwhelming evidence of the need to make room at the bedside for the pharmacist. Dispensing from the pharmacy will not provide evidence that pharmacists

have a sense of the clinical milieu, and the acceptance of the pharmacist
as an equal team member requires more than membership by fiat.

Furthermore, and this opinion was expressed by F.W.H.M. Merkus
in his inaugural editorial in Pharmacy International, pharmacists are
generally rather passive, he said, "In spite of their long university
training pharmacists refuse or hesitate to take responsibility for the
optimal use of the drugs they dispense".

Although the current emphasis on patient-orientated education
and practice appears to be having a salutary effect, mere observation of
pharmacy practice confirms the accuracy of Merkus' statement in the
majority of cases.

For social as well as for professional and economic reasons,
we have reached a point where a therapeutic team approach has gradually
become an obligation: not yet a legal obligation, however in many
situations a budgetary obligation, and definitely a moral obligation
for every professional who aspires to provide high quality health care.

We hope that the papers presented at this symposium will show
the extent to which pharmacists have overcome their traditionally somewhat passive professional behaviour, acquired new knowledge and skills
and become important members , making valuable contributions to many
therapeutic teams.

References :

DOLINSKY, D. (1982) : What is psychosocial pharmacy ?
         Pharmacy International, 33, 300 - 303.

HOOP, J. (1979) : Interprofessional Relations in Hospitals. In
         Handbook of Institutional Pharmacy Practice, ed. M.C.
         Smith and T.R. Brown, pp. 575 - 577. Baltimore :
         Williams & Wilkens.

KILWEIN, J. (1981) : Fostering a cross - cultural perspective
                     in Health care.
              Pharmacy International, 20, V - VII.

KILWEIN, J. (1982) : Science, the human condition and Pharmacy.
              Pharmacy International, 30, 202 - 204.

PROVOST, G. (1980) : The role of social and behavioral sciences in
                     pharmacy practice. Pharmacy International, 7,
                     141 - 143.

THE CONCEPT OF THE THERAPEUTIC TEAM

E. van der Kleijn,Ph.D.

Professor of Clinical Pharmacy, Catholic University of Nijmegen,Medical School, Department of Clinical Pharmacy, Sint Radboud Hospital, Geert Grooteplein Zuid 8, 6525 GA Nijmegen, the Netherlands.

Abstract

The therapeutic team concept is decribed as a practically feasible, dynamic team of physicians, nurses, pharmacists and other health professionals according to need. The team establishes the product range for drug selection,and designs calibration references for goals and objectives for treatment of patients with particular diseases, complaints or diagnoses. Therapeutic decisions still require much research on probabilities of the results. Clinical Pharmacokinetics have been helpful in establishing algorithms for decision making.

A good pharmaceutical service infrastructure in hospitals and communities with good management procedures, logistics, retrievable drug records and drug information and instruction are prerequisites for therapeutic teams

INTRODUCTION

Over 90% of patients visiting a general practitioner and of those admitted to hospitals, are prescribed drugs as the only or as support of treatment. The practice of treatment results from a decision process in which the complaints of the patients and the information, resulting from physical, anamnestic and laboratory investigation have been integrated. The complexity of diseases and of the personal variables in individuals requires coordination of expert information from different disciplines. Traditionally coordination is the task of the medical practitioner who is

consulted in first instance. Analyses of group dynamics have taught us
methods to improve the efficiency and impact of the contributions of each
expert. The financial strain on health care in the declining economy has
put more emphasis than ever in order to meet the established budgets.

A change in attitude can be observed to grant more responsibility and
executive tasks to para- or non-medical professionals in order to allow
the physician to concentrate on his expert competencies.

In several areas of chronic medical care this has been the experience for
a number of decades. Different disciplines have written information in
patients records to enable them to monitor progress. Examples are
epilepsy, diabetes, hematology and genetic diseases.

A change can be observed in the forces and powers structure of roles and
competencies and of responsibilities and liabilities in these cooperative
efforts. These social changes can also be considered consequences of the
observed necessities and of the better technical conditions for recording
and retrieving information. Prospective design of procedures and written
guidelines tailored to the various professionals involved provide
references for daily labor. Retrospective evaluation will lead to
adaptations and correction of the procedures and/or of the references.

Calibration Policy

The process of establishing references for treatment of a particular
medical indication e.g. a sub diagnosis in epilepsy requires input of
neurologists, pathologists, nurses or patient attendants, sometimes
parents, pharmacists, institution or general practice physicians, and
clerks. Establishing and continuously adjusting references for every
contributor is called 'calibration'. Daily practice is then routinely
compared, tested (titrated) against the calibre It is agreed that
intuitively many well experienced professionals will either consciously or
unconsciously comply to this process. Written procedures however make

communication easier, more stable and reliable and may allow the expertise of traditionally dispersed professionals to contribute to treatment.

General objectives for treatment and services

The patient or his attendant that made the decision to seek advice of a physician will generally want to be cured or to have his complaints resolved in a rapid, safe and effective way at the lowest expenses.

Institutions providing services to patients will try to comply to these wishes.

It is agreed today that the expenditure for National Health Care and Institutionalized care have disproportionally grown.

Governments are now seeking ways to cut on the expenses even if this should result in a lower performance level but preferably at the same quality.

In the past twelve years we have made attempts to propose and investigate ways to rationalize and economize drug selection, prescribing, preparation and dispensing, informatics, and drug documentation and consultation, monitoring and evaluation of effects in patients and of the fate of drugs in their body and drug epidemiology research (table 1).

Table 1.

Drug Selection	Formulary,Product range reduction
Prescribing	Protocols and Guidelines for treatment
Preparation	General Compounding
	I.V. admixtures
	Individualized formulation
Dispensing	Unit of use distribution
	Satellite Services
Informatics/Documentation	Management:
	Purchase
	Turn over
	Personnel Planning
	Work preparation
	Labelling
	Quality Control:
	Classification and Coding
	Batch Manufactoring Records
	Batch Distribution Records
	Scientifc Support:
	Current Awareness
	Problem solving Retrieval
	Literature Compilation
	Kinetic Analyses
Consultation	Ward rounds
	Patient conferences
	Seminars
	Symposia
Monitoring	Events registration
	Plasma concentrations and clearances
	(Clinical pharmacokinetics)
	Clinical Physiology
	Intensive Care and Emergency Medicine
Evaluation	Retrospective efforts leading to conclusions in all activities mentioned in this table.
Research	Pharmacokinetic and metabolism studies in patients and in pathological conditions
	Bio Analytical Chemistry
Drug Epidemiology	Drug Utilization Research
	Computer assisted Instruction
	Training and Instruction development.

These activities require development of organizational structures, new tools and adaptation of buildings and the training of new professionals with new knowledge, skills and attitudes.

In order to keep these activities economically feasible management decisions at different levels are required.

Product range reduction

Structural improvement on hospital and community level can be expected from product range reduction Formulary- or Pharmacy and Therapeutics Committees have proven their beneficial effect of the voluntary acceptance of compulsory recommendations on product selection. It can be expected that this will gradually lead to a 10-20% reduction in drug expenditure with the risk that when the compulsory nature of choice restriction is not well executed tensions and frustrations develop leading to reduction of initial achievements (1).

Drug utilization recommendations

Retrospective analysis of the use of drugs on individual, ward, hospital, regional, national and international level can diligently alert increases and decreases in use. It can be useful when steep increases are observed to call for 'ad hoc' expert consensus committees to design guidelines and protocols for the appropriate and economic use of groups of drugs. In general one will attack the expensive and most frequently used drugs or drug groups such as albumin, antibiotics, perfusion solutions etc.(2.3.4).

Calibration

The attendance of different professionals in the ad hoc committee often is difficult to maintain after the recommendations have been accepted and implemented. Ad hoc committees generally operate at hospital level and their effects lacks the personal committment.

Calibration, a well accepted term in pharmacy is meant here as a term that is also applicable in medicine as reference for the contribution of every professional in the therapeutic team. The references can prospectively be established and tested, be used in daily practice and can retrospectively be evaluated and adapted.

Successful approaches have been reported in epilepsy (5) in infectious diseases (6) Oncology (7),and Parenteral nutrition (4) The tasks and responsibilities of every member can be defined leading to acceptance of each other competencies. The term audit practiced as an intercollegeal effort focusses on the quality of the care rather than the quantity. Budgetting is now used by hospital managers but the suspicion of the medical community remains that this term focusses on the quantitative, economic, objectives rather than on quality (figure 1).

Schematic expression of the various terms used in hospital politics to balance quality of care and quantity of expenditure.

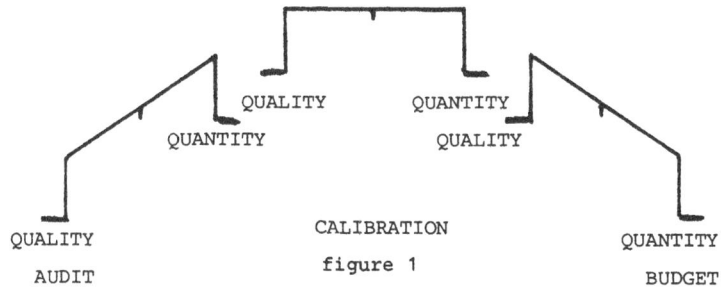

QUALITY
QUANTITY

QUANTITY
QUALITY

QUALITY
AUDIT

CALIBRATION
figure 1

QUANTITY
BUDGET

Therapeutic decision making

The motives leading to the selection of a particular treatment following the decision of the most likely diagnosis are often complex and not seldom intuitive. Several approaches have been suggested to improve on the reliability, the probability and confidence of the intended outcome of a chosen therapy or therapeutic(8).

Algorithms are well layed out analyses of the sequential steps leading to desired effects. Decision trees can be constructed so each branch can theoretically lead to this result. At the bifurcation points that are moments of decision, statistical probabilities will support the likelihood of the desired effect. These algorithms can be useful tools for a calibration team in order to establish the recommendations and tasks of the members(6).

Concluding remarks

The therapeutic team concept is described as a scientific and economic necessity, and an organizational requirement for the maintenance of good quality care.

The pharmacists' contribution can be viewed from his traditional role as a drug manufacturer, dispenser and consultant and from his more recently acquired knowledge, skills and attitude in therapeutics and pharmacokinetics (figure 2).

In particular the recent contributions of clinical pharmacokinetics to the decision making of therapeutics, allows an important role of the pharmacists in clinical toxicology, therapeutic drug monitoring, development of selection criteria e.g. by establishing probabilities, and last but not least research in drug and pathology related variables in patients and in volunteers.

Schematic position of the therapeutic team of physician, nurse and clinical pharmacokinetically trained professional that can coordinate questions and needs of the patient, the team members and the pharmacy.

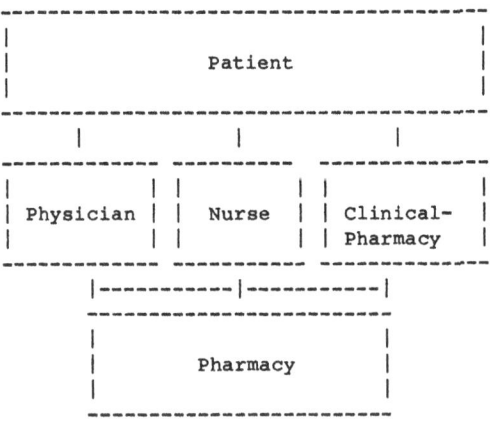

figure 2

REFERENCES

1.Kleijn, van der E.,Hekster, Y.A., Zuidgeest,L.B.J., Janssen, W.,and
  Termond,E.(1981) Economic and therapeutic consequences of voluntary
  drug product range and consumption reduction. In Drug
  Utilization Studies in Hospitals, eds. Dr. M. Hollmann,
  Prof.Dr.E.Weber.13-22,F.K.Schattauer Verlag, Stuttgart-New York.

2.Hekster,Y.A.,Goris, R.J.A., Lamers, C.B.H.,and Kleijn, van der, E.,
  Influence of guidelines on the utilization pattern of plasma
  protein and albumin. (1979) In. Progress of Clinical Pharmacy.
  eds. D. Schaaf and E. van der Kleijn, 229-234. Elsevier/North Holland
  Biomedical Press.

3.Hekster,Y.A.,Goris, J.,Boerema,H., Zuidgeest,T.Smeekens,T.,
  Friesen,W. and Kleijn, van der,E., Effects of audit on drug utilization
  patterns in a hospital. In. Progress of Clinical Pharmacy III, Eds.
  H. Turakka and E. van der Kleijn (1981) 141-151.Elsevier/North Holland
  Biomedical Press, Amsterdam, New York, Oxford.

4.Nguyen Ung Tach, Bakker, H., Zuidgeest,T. and Kleijn, van der, E.
  Investigation of the consumption of parenteral solutions of large
  volume and other selected sterile fluids in the Sint Radboud Hospital.
  In Progress In Clinical Pharmacy II,(1980)237-245. Eds. J.C.Plasse and
  E. van der Kleijn. Elsevier/North Holland Biomedical Press.Amsterdam,
  New York, Oxford.

5.Schobben,A.F.A.M., Vingerhoets,D., Cremers, M.,Essen van C. and Kleijn
  van der, E. The rationalisation of therapy in institution. In The
  Rational Prescribing of Antiepileptic Drug. S. Shorvon et al.,eds. in
  press.

6.Hekster, Y.A. (1983) Selection criteria for Antimicrobial Drug
  Utilization,Thesis, Nijmegen.

7.Kleijn, van der, E., Vree, T.B., Oosterbaan,M., and Schobben,F.(1982)
  Clinical Pharmacokinetics in the therapeutic management of patients. In
  Pharmacokinetics a Modern View. Eds. G. Levy and L.Z. Benet,Plenum
  Publ. Company. New York, in press.

8.Weinstein,M.C., Fineberg,H.V.(1980) Clinical Decision Analysis,
  W.B. Saunders Company, Philadelphia, London, Toronto.

THE THERAPEUTIC TEAM CONCEPT - THE VIEW OF A PHARMACIST.

J.P. Delporte
Pharmacy Institute, University of Liège, rue Fusch, 5,
4000 Liège, Belgium.

Definition and main applications

The therapeutic team (T.T.) concept may be defined as an
association of varied and complementary competences, responsibilities and
activities through which the physician, pharmacist and nurse aim mainly
at reaching a better well-being of the patient and the correct use of
drugs. These objectives are essentially realized through the following
activities :

- drug therapy selection, application and survey;
- development and improvement of therapeutic techniques;
- establishment of guidelines on procedures or material use
  and selection;
- information and education.

What seems fundamental for the pharmacist is the new part he
can play in the T.T. In fact, the ultimate objective of the pharmacist
is no longer the drug itself, its preparation, control, storage and
distribution, but rather the "drug-patient" relationship he can concretely
develop through different patient-oriented tasks :

- presence in patient care areas and patient rounds with the
  physician
- patient interview and establishment of medication history;
- medication, administration route and form selection or
  counseling;
- drug preparation and sometimes administration;
- posology control and drug monitoring;
- prevention of drug interactions (drug-drug, drug-food,
  drug-lab test interactions) and contraindications;
- treatment survey and drug side-effect detection;
- physician, nurse or patient information and education.

The integration of the pharmacist in most of these applications seems to be less and less contested and is even becoming to be considered a necessity. On the other hand, the limits of his intervention are much more controversial with the result that the manner and degree of integration of the pharmacist into the T.T. is often very different depending on the country or the hospital itself. That is why presently the T.T. concept is still an imprecise notion to which everyone is tempted to give his own definition.

Clinical activities evolution

Nowhere **have clinical** pharmacy services developed so deeply as in the USA. In many hospitals - currently about 25 % of American hospitals have developed a clinical program - the clinical pharmacist is permanently present in patient care areas : he makes patient rounds, consults with the medical staff, takes part in decisions on drug therapy or the necessity of extending or interrupting hospital treatment, helps the patient to treat his own disease, etc...

Such an integration of the clinical pharmacist in the T.T. requires more and more specific knowledge and very specialized education and training markedly oriented to a defined field of medecine. In this way he is becoming a subspecialist in oncology, cardiology, psychiatry,... so that we may sometimes meet 30 or 40 of them distributed throughout the different medical or surgical services. In fact clinical pharmacy services are being set up in most areas of medicine : psychiatry, pediatry, cardiology, cardio-pulmonary and post-surgery recovery, oncology, TPN, radiopharmacy, rehabilitation center, ...without taking into account internal medical subdivisions where clinical pharmacists are sometimes only concerned with specific problems : anticoagulant therapy, diabetes, hypertension, geriatry, etc..., for inpatients as well as for outpatients. In the USA, this subspecialisation has induced the mushrooming of clinical pharmacy services and some clinical pharmacists would prefer to remain independent of the pharmacy and its distribution function. This we can judge from the content of recent editorials and publications in the American Journal of Hospital Pharmacy (ZELLMER, 1981, SCHNEIDER, 1981).

The development of clinical pharmacy programs in this country has certainly enjoyed great success thanks to different motivating factors the most decisive of which was, and probably still is, the scarcity of nurses. This parameter alone has justified the presence of the pharmacist

in the patient care area and opened the doors wide for the setting up of
satellite pharmacies. By simultaneously solving the problem of
communication, these decentralized pharmacies establish much more
credibility in the relationship between the pharmacist and the medical
staff.

Of course, other parameters have contributed to promote
clinical pharmacy : medication errors, specific and complementary
education programs for physicians and pharmacists, the need for more
organized drug information, new therapeutic techniques, the advent of
biopharmacy and pharmacokinetics, and also another necessary incentive
parameter : more facilities for reimbursement of clinical pharmaceutical
expenditure.

In Europe, in spite of an increasing number of important
applications in the field of clinical pharmacy service, it should be
emphasized that these activities are evolving more slowly and in more
isolated instances. Whereas a few pharmacists have effectively
implemented large clinical programs, others have undertaken only limited
or spontaneous activities. For example, in our old university and public
health hospital of Liège, a few activities, greatly appreciated by the
medical staff, have been developed requiring the collaboration of
everyone, physician, pharmacist and nurse, in TPN, extracorporeal and
peritoneal dialysis, oncological I.V. solution preparation, the search
for efficient methods of disinfection, etc...

In the current economic situation however, how many
well-intentioned efforts have not been discouraged by innumerous
hindrances : existing legal requirements, poorly motivated environment,
over-conventional conceptions, unadapted education, financial
restrictions,lack of understanding and the insufficient long-term
prospective view of public health financing organisations?

Towards priority objectives

Under these conditions and in the disastrous financial
situation of our hospitals, we are convinced that clinical pharmacy in
Europe must implement ways not necessarily copied from "the American
model" for it is unreasonable to try and perform, with a ratio of one
pharmacist for 150, 200 or even 400 beds, the same activities accomplished
elsewhere with one pharmacist for 15 or 30 beds.

We are therefore obliged to look for other working methods and determine priorities depending on our human, technical and financial capacities. To this end, we must concentrate our efforts on tasks which have every chance of success, i.e. those which appear necessary rather than simply interesting complementary measures.

Priority programs will obviously be those that will be revealed as profitable in so far as patient health is concerned, and those that will harmoniously and complementarily make use of the specific competences and education of those involved. Several surveys carried out in the USA have clearly revealed that all activities which may put the pharmacist in a conflicting position with the physician do not generally succeed. On the other hand, physicians often ask for closer cooperation in fields where pharmacist competency is much more involved : prescription control (posology, interactions,...), drug monitoring, drug profile maintenance, information etc...(KELLY & SEAVER, 1981, RITCHEY & RANEY, 1981, SCHNEIDER, 1981, MALLETT, 1982).

Ways of reaching priority objectives

The right drug, in the right dose, at the right time, for the right patient. Although simply defined, this first objective of clinical pharmacists nevertheless covers a wide clinical program.

A lot of drug distribution systems have been designed to achieve this objective to a greater or lesser degree, some based on a centralized and individualized distribution in the central pharmacy, others on the setting up of peripheral distribution stations, satellite pharmacies or stocks on the wards. Is one of these systems better than the others? Certainly not since there is no reference system. The best systems are those which are well adapted to the particular hospital situation and local circumstances : available man-power, hospital architecture and substructure, financial situation etc... Nevertheless, in the current economic context in Belgium, the setting up of satellite pharmacies is a difficult, maybe impossible challenge. It is more realistic to organize a distribution system, either decentralized but relying on a much closer and continuous cooperation with the physician and above all the nurse (the system established by VAN DER KUY in the Tilburg hospitals is a specially representative model), or centralized but efficiently solving the problem of communication between the pharmacy and the patient care areas. In this field, the use of computers will force itself upon us as an increasingly indispensable tool. To ignore this would be a gross error.

Under pressure of financial difficulties, the Maine Medical Center in Portland has developed one of the most computerized hospital management systems in the USA, establishing a permanent communication between the central pharmacy and patient care areas by means of VDU terminals. This system permits the efficient transfer of physician prescriptions and their modifications, posology and interaction controls, day-to-day maintenance of the drug profile, the printing of non-equivocal work sheets for the pharmacist (drug distribution sheets, I.V. solution prescription sheets,...) and for the nurse (administration record sheets), not to mention many further possibilities in the field of management, invoicing, drug use statistics, etc...(GOUSSE, 1978).

Taking over routine and administrative management functions, a computerized system makes the pharmacist more available for clinical tasks and presence in patient care areas.

Whatever the adopted drug distribution system may be, two minimal conditions are required to meet the defined objectives :

- first, the pharmacist must always be able to check the physician 's prescription;

- second, he must be able to check the dispensed medications, survey their effects on the patient, especially by maintaining the access to the patient 's medical record. The clinical pharmacist may thus efficiently contribute to drug use survey programs.

As far as medication distribution itself and the uncontested value of unit dose is concerned we must recognise that up to now in Europe, efforts have been mainly focused on oral dosage forms which are the most widely used in hospital practice but do not present as high therapeutical and toxicological risks as I.V. solutions.

Since the setting up of a 24 hours-a-day centralized I.V. additive operating service like in a few American hospital pharmacies creates almost insurmountable obstacles here, our intervention must therefore be more spontaneous and selective. A few clinical pharmacists have well realized this necessity and devoted all their efforts to the preparation in the central pharmacy and in the best conditions only of higher-risk I.V. fluids : TPN solutions, chemotherapy I.V. solutions and emergency medications in prefilled syringes rather than in multidose vials.

The even partial handling of I.V. solutions by the pharmacist will be all the more efficient as it will lead to the development of systematic and organized information for the nurse, enabling her to take responsibility for the I.V. fluids that the pharmacy do not take in charge. To this end, two precautionary measures may be recommended:

- each I.V. solution admixture must be ordered on detailed and clear prescription sheets and be submitted to the supervising pharmacist prior to mixing so that he can alert the nurse to any special problems;

- formulary drug-product monographs must contain guidelines for the handling and administration of certain I.V. medications.

Furthermore, information is another priority objective to which the clinical pharmacist has to apply himself. To the numerous daily information demands he receives, he must provide quick and precise answers otherwise he will lose credibility. Particular attention must be devoted to this task and its importance has been demonstrated in the USA by the creation of information centers solely devoted to this function.

The nature of questions usually raised (SCHWEIGERT, OPPENHEIMER & SMITH, 1982, BABINGTON, ROBINSON & MONSON, 1982) indicates however that without organizing so highly specialized centers, the pharmacist already has efficient means at his disposal to divulge information and respond to a large number of requests, particulary through the formulary and via therapeutic and hygiene committees.

Complementary to a restrictive list of freely available medications, a carefully conceived formulary may constitute a valuable source of information on drugs : identification, dose, posology, indications, contraindications, administration route, stability, storage, interactions, etc... In the same way, within the different committees, the pharmacist takes part in the elaboration of guidelines for drug or sterile material selection and in the establishment of working procedures (drug or sterile material handling, disinfection techniques,...) and in general for anything that concerns the patient's health. Besides this consultative work is another way to learn of the problems raised in the wards.

In this presentation, I have limited myself to a few aspects of the pharmacist's integration into the T.T. Let us point out however that, to develop clinical activities, is not the sole purpose as it is valuable only where it aims at patient's health and security. The energy devoted by the clinical pharmacist would thus be useless if it had no extension outside the hospital. For example, the advantages of a decrease in the use of antibiotics in the hospital would be incomplete if the same efforts were not extended to ambulatory medicine. A dialogue and a close collaboration must therefore be maintained between medico-pharmaceutical sectors inside and outside the hospital.

In conclusion, I am convinced that any sufficiently motivated hospital pharmacist, acting within his abilities, can now combine different clinical activities within the actual structures of our hospital pharmaceutical organisation. Anyone, no matter the size of the hospital he is working for, disposes or may dispose of means to start or develop a closer collaboration with the physician and the nurse, either in vast clinical programs or in more spontaneous interventions.

Finally, the T.T. must not be seen only as the concentration of people with different competences within very limited confines, but as a communion of thoughts and efforts oriented towards the better well-being of the patient and the correct use of drugs.

Reference list

Babington M.A., Robinson T.A., Monson R.A., A.J.H.P., (1982), 39, 127-8.
Covinsky J.O., (1979), in Handbook of Institutional Pharmacy Practice
    ed. M.C. Smith and T.R. Brown, Williams & Wilkins, London, 472-8.
Gousse W.L., A.J.H.P., (1978), 35, 711-4.
Kelly W.N. & Seaver D.J., A.J.H.P., (1981), 38, 1786-8.
Mallett M.S., A.J.H.P., (1982), 39, 410-1.
Ritchey F.J. & Raney M.R., A.J.H.P., (1981), 38, 1459-63.
Schneider P.J., A.J.H.P., (1981), 38, 1784-6.
Schweigert B.F., Oppenheimer P.R. & Smith W.E., A.J.H.P., (1982), 39, 74-7.
Smith W.E. & Mackevicz D.W. (1979), in Handbook of Institutional Pharmacy
    Practice, ed. M.C. Smith and T.R. Brown, Williams & Wilkins,
    Baltimore-London, 465-71.
Zellmer W.A., A.J.H.P., (1981), 38, 177.

THE CONCEPT OF THE THERAPEUTIC TEAM : VIEW OF A PHYSICIAN

M.G. Bogaert
Heymans Institute of Pharmacology, University of Gent Medical
School, B-9000 Gent, Belgium

Discussions about the role of the clinical pharmacist in the therapeutic team tend to be rather emotional, and it is far from easy to define this role. One should therefore try to make things somewhat easier, by looking at an answer to this question in function of the hospital where the clinical pharmacist is working, of the training of the clinical pharmacist involved and of the presence or absence of physicians trained in pharmacology and pharmacokinetics.

Physicians certainly expect from the clinical pharmacist factual information about the drugs available in the hospital. Indeed, physicians are often faced with problems such as generic versus trade names, possible substitutes for a product no longer available, etc.

Information about possible interactions and possible side-effects of newer and older drugs should also be available at the hospital pharmacy. The availability of this information can be coupled with an attempt to organise a feed-back system concerning interactions and side-effects. Most physicians will appreciate that somebody is able to draw their attention to the fact that two drugs they have prescribed together, can give rise to a potentially dangerous interaction, which was not known to the physician or which he had overlooked. And even if the physician was well aware of the drug interaction, and in fact had decided that the possible danger is outweighed by the expected benefit to the patient, a warning by the pharmacist should not unduly worry the physician.

In order to make such a system workable, the clinical pharmacist has to have a good knowledge about interactions which goes beyond the availability of endless lists. It is indeed of importance that the clinical pharmacist is able to distinguish between all possible or ever described interactions, and those which have a chance to elicit a clinically relevant problem. Otherwise the collaboration will certainly not last.

Whether or not it is useful that the pharmacist comes to the bedside in order to detect or discuss interactions and side-effects, or compliance, can be debated. Most physicians, at least in our country, do not expect the pharmacist to do that. One could argue that this is not logical, as physicians themselves do not give enough time to side-effects, interactions, compliance. But the clinical pharmacist should not only be interested in those things that other people do not find the time to do or are not willing to do and one should try to find out who is best equipped to handle these things. For many of them one does not need to be a physician or a pharmacist, and a nurse will probably function better e.g. for detection of side-effects or interactions.

In regard to questioning the patient, the clinical pharmacist will often be at a disadvantage. Indeed he is usually not trained in clinical medicine or pathophysiology. And understanding what is happening to a patient in renal failure, or to a patient with a complex interaction, does not only involve knowledge of the properties of the drug but also knowledge of the way the body functions and of what is wrong in the organism of this particular patient.

Therefore one should not try to split up the patients' problem as if diagnosis and decision to treat belong to the physician and choice of the drug, dosage etc., to the pharmacist. Both physician and pharmacist will function better if they collaborate.

Many clinical pharmacists are involved in the field of drug monitoring and clinical pharmacokinetics. This is not unexpected as the training of a pharmacist prepares him well for the analytical aspects, while for organisational purposes, in many hospitals the analysis is done within the framework of the hospital pharmacy. This is certainly in many places a satisfactory arrangement. But here again what the physician expects from the pharmacist will certainly be different from hospital to hospital. If clinical pharmacologists or pharmacologists with interest in the matter are available, they also should be involved in drug monitoring and clinical pharmacokinetics, e.g. in collaboration with the clinical pharmacist. Indeed for interpretation of the plasma concentration of a drug, knowledge of the physiological processes and more particularly of the pathophysiological processes e.g. in renal failure, a hepatic disease is needed.

One could argue that a clinical pharmacist could try to learn about the physiopathology and about clinical medicine so that he is able to function properly, without the need for collaboration with physicians, e.g. for interpretation of results of plasma concentration assays. This is certainly not very efficient, and one cannot expect that a clinical pharmacist gains this knowledge by doing some reading on the subject.

It is clear that pharmacists and physicians function best if they try to help each other on the basis of the particular knowledge they possess.

It is not easy to define these respective roles and they will certainly be very different from country to country and from hospital to hospital, depending upon the expertise of the persons involved.

THE CONCEPT OF THE THERAPEUTIC TEAM. THE VIEW OF A NURSE

M. Michiels
University Hospital St Rafaël, Capucynenvoer 35, 3000
Louvain, Belgium

INTRODUCTION: THE HOSPITAL PHARMACIST AND THE NURSE

In the hospital pharmacists and nurses have mutual responsibilities and expectations. However none of the parties ever mentions these expectations.

In the following exposition I'll try to make a proposal which integrates both patterns of expectations.

I'll start with a definition of both professions:

"Clinical pharmacy is a health-science specialty, whose responsibility it is to assure the safe and appropriate use of drugs in patients through the application of specialized knowledge and functions in patient care, and which necessitates specialized education and/or structured training. It requires use of judgment in the collection and interpretation of data, patient specific involvement and direct interprofessional interaction." (Committee on Clinical Pharmacy as a Specialty, Minnesota, November 15, 1981)

"The unique function of the nurse exists in supporting the individual (healthy or ill) by doing activities that contribute to the health or recovery and that should be done by the individual itself if he or she should have enough power energy or knowledge. The nurse has to perform this task in such a way that the patient should become independant as soon as possible." (according to Florence Nightingale, Virginia Henderson, Dorothy Hall ...)

Nursing is a science, being a combination of separate sciences as physical, medical and social sciences, and an art by applying those sciences in practice. It supposes a systematic, purposeful and well considered way of acting, described in the literature as 'systematic nursing action'.

As can be concluded from both definitions clinical pharmacy

and nursing are both involved in patient care. Conflicts are difficult
to   avoid   when the action field of both professions is not well
defined.

However both having their typical functions the point of
view of a nurse is obvious:"The nurses do the nursing, other persons do
not the nursing".

1: THE HOSPITAL PHARMACIST AND THE NURSE WORKING
AS A TEAM

In the past only physician and nurse were mentioned when
talking about patient care. Meanwhile different other people have joined
those two; psychologists, social workers, physical therapeutists and
others.

It's strange that almost nobody mentions pharmacists. Why
not?

I think the reason is we have to differentiate between:-
- direct patient care executed by the people mentioned above
- indirect patient care where the pharmacist is involved.

2: RELATION BETWEEN HOSPITAL PHARMACIST AND NURSE
FROM MY OWN EXPERIENCE

In our hospital I work in three kinds of fields:
hospitalisation wards, operating-rooms and the committee on hospital
hygiene.

I'll give a review of my experiences in these fields.

2.1. The committee on hospital hygiene

In this committee pharmacist is recognized because of his
knowledge acquired by study and experience. Experts are talking to
each other in a direct interprofessional relationship.

I'll give some examples that illustrate the good cooperation
between pharmacist and the other members of the committee.

2.1.1. First Example

The manual of hospital hygienics, being three years old,
had to be reviewed. We seized the opportunity to revise the whole
package of disinfectants according to their use and efficacy.

We were happy we could call on pharmacist to give us some
ideas about:

a. The different disinfectants used and their annual
turnover

b. The stability of solutions

c. The possible incompatibilities

d. The packing of disinfectants, bearing in mind the packing
charges.

2.1.2. Second Example

Several nurses complained about injuries caused when breaking
glass ampoules. Under the supervision of the committee a study,
coordinated by the pharmacist, was carried out about the use of plastic
ampoules.

Personally I enjoy the good cooperation between the different
members of the committee. I think it is a result of the professional
way we're working. But most of all it is an organized form of
communication,respected and even encouraged by the hospital directors.

2.2. The operating-rooms

From my personal experience I can tell there 's a good
cooperation between pharmacy and nursing in the operating-rooms.
From pharmacy nurses expect especially:

- An easy identification of drugs. E.g. the pharmacist
  contacted the manufacturers to have a clear distinction
  made between different ampoules.
- Information about industrially manufactured sterile sets.
  The pharmacist is the ideal person between the manufacturer and the nursing. And he's best placed to inform
  the nursing about new kinds of sets.
- Information about drug incompatibilities especially in
  infusion liquids.
- Cooperation with the pharmacist when doing clinical trials
  with new drugs, e.g. anesthetics.

The pharmacist, on his side, shall try to keep stocks in
the operating-rooms as low as possible. He shall insist to register
any drug and material used. The primary reason being a financial one,
this attitude, however, also brings on a limitation of the drug use
and a rational prescribing by the physicians.

In contrast with the committee on hospital hygiene in the
case of the operating-rooms there is no organized network of
communication. Nor is there for the hospitalisation wards. In part 3
I'll try to make a proposal in that direction.

2.3. The hospitalisation wards

Physician, nurse and pharmacist, all of them want to give
to the patient a right medication. But their approximation to the
problem is quite different. Let us consider their respective expectations:

a. The nurse

- Expects that drugs are available as soon as possible.
- Prefers unit dose.
- Expects measures to prevent drug interactions.
- Doesn't like to much administrative work.
- Expects information from the pharmacist:

- about new drugs
- about price and **reimbursement** of drugs
- about side-effects of drugs for patient and
  for nurse (e.g. cytotoxic drugs)
- about what has to be done when discharging the
  patient.

b. The pharmacist

- Expects the original prescription and an insight in the
  total therapy.
- Expects an almost faultless drug distribution system, that
  keep stocks on the wards as small as possible. The number
  of drugs should be limited by a drug formulary.
- Expects that drugs will be prescribed conscious of their
  price.

c. The physician

- Expects that will be executed what he has prescribed.
- Expects no administrative work.
- Expects that nurse and pharmacist will rectify obvious
  errors in his prescriptions.

All three of them want to push through their own expectations. So it's obvious that an agreement only can be reached after
mutual consultation with respect for the different fields of action.

But let us not forget that the last link in giving medication
to the patient is the nurse: the nurse has a strategic position to judge
the value of a drug distribution system.

If somebody asks me if pharmacist should be involved in the
therapeutic team, then my answer will be positive. But I cannot agree
with the pharmacist giving the drug to the patient. Because
giving medication is but one action in a total of actions, as e.g.
controling the drip chamber of an infusion set, measuring temperature,
controle of blood pressure. And these actions shall be done by the nurse.

I conclude: Nurse and pharmacist have both a unique and
autonomous function in health care, both having their own **responsi-**
bilities. However, they are dependant on each-other as grown-up members
of the health-care-team.

3: PROPOSAL OF INTEGRATION

One has to come to a cooperation between both parties, when they work with appreciation and respect for each other. Because appreciation and respect for the patient suppose appreciation and respect between all parties that take care of him.

This also means that one respects the expert knowledge and the capacities of the others and complements these with his/her own expertise. This professional attitude only can grow by interprofessional interaction with   excellent communication.

Communication means that one communicates the data that are relevant to the other. E.g. important drug interactions.

Communication also means that all parties discuss the problems. Even when one cannot find a solution to his problem, it is good to know that one has not to face his problem alone.

This attitude of respect, interest and communication asks for flexible people and not for rigid positions. It is necessary to be open for new insights and to be prepared to keep on looking for a human response to the needs of the patient.

Nurses have a special function in this team, because they are on the bedside of the patient during twenty-four hours. They can play the important role of coordinator of all the services for their patients.

The physician in charge of the pain clinic e.g. relies on to a great extent on the information received from the nursing. Indeed:

- who can control better the side-effects of the drugs?

- who can answer better the question if the patient tolerates the treatment?

- who will first find out if a patient abuses a drug?

- who observes better the patient, when he is taken off the drug?

- who can better talk to the patient and give him all the information he needs?

- who knows better the personal facts of the patient?

A team approach is very important in this matter. But what is the position of the pharmacist in this team?

When a physician starts his treatment, the nurse is aware

of the side effects. When nobody takes care of the patient and doesn't look to his medication properly, it can be dangerous to patients health.

From the observations of the nurse, given to the physician and to the pharmacist, the drug can be withdrawn and replaced by another.

One has also to consider the two nursing systems: primary nursing and team nursing. Primary nursing means that one nurse receives the responsibility for one patient from admission to discharge. Team nursing means that a team of nurses receive the responsibility for a whole group of patients.

However, whether one practices primary nursing or team nursing or whatever the system may be, the cooperation between a nurse and a pharmacist can function properly.

What system can be proposed now on the basis of all these considerations?

- Do we have to consider the implementation of 'nurse observers?
- Do we have to reorganize the set-up of a nursing station? The pharmacist comes up to the floor and discusses the problems with the nursing or with the head nurse.
- Do we have to consider the formation of a new committee with an identical structure as the mentioned committee on hospital hygiene?, the pharmacist being a member of a pharmacy and therapeutics committee where he discusses the problems with a delegate of the nursing and a delegate of the physicians.

For every system however we need respect and appreciation between the team members and the approval of the hospital administration.

Every system has its advantages and disadvantages. One system cannot be proposed, because a lot depends on the capacities of each team member and the characteristics of the hospital, government regulations, etc.

Personally I decide in favour of the committee for pharmacy and therapeutics. I don't think there is time to discuss problems with the pharmacy by telephone for every nurse. Maybe these questions can be written down on a special form sheet, collected and sent to the pharmacy of course. I don't want to exclude the physicians, who are an exponent of our interprofessional relationship.

The key of the operation of a therapeutic team is the personality of each team member. Besides their intellectual capacities they need to have an ability to communicate with others.

REFERENCES

Armstrong-esther (C.A.), Standards of nursing-care, Nursing Times, January 1, 1981, vol. 77, 1

Clifford J.C., Primary nursing: a contemporary model for delivery of care, American Journal of Hospital Pharmacy, vol 37, aug. 1981

Gourley (D.R.), Integrating pharmaceutical services and education in an academic medical center, American Journal of Hospital Pharmacy, vol. 39, jan 1982

Hall (D.C.), Position paper an nursing, Copenhagen, WHO, Regional Office for Europe, EURO/NURS/75.1., 1975,p.1

Henderson (V.), Grondbeginselen van de verpleegkunde, De Tijdstroom, Lochem, 1976

Keirse (M.), De apotheker: begeleider voor zieke en gezin, Academische Ziekenhuizen, K.U.Leuven

Maulsch (I.G.), Nurse-physician collaboration: a changing relationship, The Journal of Nursing Administration,june 1981

Mc Nutt Devereux (P), Essential elements of nurse-physician collaboration, The Journal of Nursing Administration, may 1981

Mc Nutt Devereux (P.), Does joint practice work?, The Journal of Nursing Administration, June 1981

Montesinos (A.), De verpleegkundige en de organisatie van het ziekenhuiswerk, De Tijdstroom, 1976

Morato (L.), Nursing compliance in the hospital, Hospital de la Sta. Cruz, Barcelona, Spain

Rogers (A.G.), Psychosocial and nursing technique, Advances in pain research and therapy, vol. 2, edited by J.J. Bonica and V. Ventafridda, Raven Press, New York, 1979

Schotfeldt (R.M.), Nursing and clinical pharmacy, Cleveland Ohio, Elsevier, 1977

Schweigert (B.F.), Hospital pharmacists as a source of drug

information for physicians and nurse, American Journal of
 Hospital Pharmacy, vol. 39, jan. 1982

Stolar (M.H.), Pharmacy—coordinated investigations drug
services, American Journal of Hospital Pharmacy, vol. 39,
1982

Stolte (J.B.), Zieken en hun verzorgers, H.D. Tjeen Willink,
Groningen, 1976

THE THERAPEUTIC TEAM. THE VIEW OF A CLINICAL PHARMACOLOGIST.

Dr.D.M.Chaput de Saintonge,
Department of Pharmacology and Therapeutics,
London Hospital Medical College,
Turner Street,
London, E1 2AD

As a clinical pharmacologist I have a special interest in and
responsibility for optimising drug treatment for each individual patient.
One component of this concerns the ideal use of the therapeutic team to
achieve the most efficient treatment of patients. By training and
inclination I stand at the interface between clinical pharmacy and
medicine so it is with the interaction between them that I will be most
concerned in this paper. However I would like to emphasise that many
of the points of principle that I will make could be applied to any
professional interface either within the therapeutic team or outside
medicine entirely. I must also say my point of view is entirely
personal and is not intended to represent the view of clinical pharmacology in the U.K.

It would be unnecessary for me to promote the need for a
team approach to medical treatment to the current audience; particularly
its need in the context of the conditions to be discussed in later papers.
I must however point out that the most important member of the team has
not yet been allowed to speak here. He is, of course, the patient
himself. In the vast majority of occasions on which drugs are given
the patient is the only member of the team and takes on the roles of all
the others. Even when the full team is present and active, the
patient may still choose the other members and sanction their actions by
his compliance with their advice (or otherwise). The extent to which
the patient actually dominates the therapeutic team varies according to
the medical problem, and the setting in which it occurs. However I
believe it is important for efficient and harmonious team relationships
for us all to remember that the whole structure is, or should be,
patient-centred. The team exists to provide an optimal solution to the

patient's problem.   This does not mean only that the patient supplies the problem, nor even that his views about what constitutes an optimal solution are relevant (which of course they are).   It also means that each member of the team has a professional responsibility to the patient, and this should override the financial, emotional and intra-professional pressures which all too often compromise the integrity of team-work in the Health Service.

From my highly- biased point of view as a clinical pharmacologist I would like to look at some of the relationships between pharmacy and medicine, concentrating on the factors which lead to suboptimal judgments about drug treatment.   I will also try to suggest some ways in which the making of these judgments might be improved.   In this I am heavily indebted to Professor Ken Hammond from the Institute of Behavioral Science in Boulder, Colorado, who is responsible for the development of much of this way of looking at the resolution of conflict in human judgment.   But please do not hold him responsible for the things I am going to say now!

Our roles and their relationships within the therapeutic team are governed by a number of factors, some of them alterable, others beyond our control.   Among those relevant to the present problem are:-

Personal intellectual, emotional and social characteristics which lead us to select a particular type and place of work.   Some of these may be the result of long exposure to certain work pressures, but it seems likely that most are factors which determine our preference for, and possibly our suitability for, one professional role rather than another.   Our emotional needs to be valued by society and our fellow professionals will also influence our choice of jobs and how we respond to the actions and attitudes of other team members.   Training provides the knowledge, skills and some of the professional attitudes necessary for us to maintain our roles effectively.   Some of this training will reflect tradition in that at the core of every professional training is an area which, by virtue of many years continued practice, is thought of as indisputably exclusive 'territory'.   However, even such traditional practices can be eroded, for instance in the way the pharmaceutical industry has taken over many of the manufacturing and dispensing functions traditionally within the domain of the pharmacist.   Such outside pressures create strong forces for action and reaction within professions, but not necessarily for the good of their clients.   It is the patients'

needs which should be creating the strongest pressures for modifying
attitudes and behaviour within and between members of the therapeutic
team.

Let us now look at a few of the traditional activities of
doctors and pharmacists and see how we might classify the judgments they
involve.   Pharmacists firstly dispense and prepare special formulations
according to established procedures.   Taken at a superficial level this
involves no element of judgment, the procedure being precisely laid down
and the pharmacist having a fine degree of control over the variables
which might influence the nature of the final product.   Secondly,
pharmacists are responsible for quality control of some manufactured
products from which they may take a sample for testing dissolution or
disintegration rates.   Here the judgment that quality is acceptable rests
on extrapolation from the results of tests on the sample.   Scientific
methods involving standard sampling techniques and accepted modes of
statistical inference allow such judgments to be made with a defined level
of confidence.   A third type of activity requiring a greater degree of
judgment by the pharmacist concerns the selection of generic equivalents.
Here the pharmacist rarely experiments himself but relies on published
data from various sources, some of which is of a comparative nature, some
of which is not.   From this he decides which brand of that drug would be
appropriate for use in a population which may never have been represented
in the studies which formed the basis for the decision.   Judgments of
this type are open to question in ways which the first two were not
because the pharmacist now has little power to manipulate conditions but
must select data from the observations of others by using his own judgment.
An even greater degree of judgment is required in monitoring prescriptions
for safety.   Here the pharmacist is given some items of data such as the
drugs and their doses, and then decides whether the prescription is safe
to dispense.   His judgment is aided by knowledge of some rules or
principles relating to undesirable drug combinations, optimal dosing
frequency and the normal range of drug doses.   Notice that there is no
element of experiment or testing here and that the pharmacist's judgment
of a prescription's safety cannot rest on any prospective observations in
that patient.

The four levels of activity by the pharmacist we have considered involve a steadily decreasing degree of control over the environment
and the data it provides and an increasing substitution of what is called

human judgment. Traditionally many therapeutic decisions by doctors
seem to start at the other end of the scale. For example, general
practitioners' decisions to prescribe antibiotics are often made on the
grounds that the patient 'needs them'. Much human judgment probably
proceeds at this level. When exercised by doctors it is politely called
'clinical opinion' and its value sanctioned by 'clinical experience'.
Such judgments may prove to be quite correct but as pronouncements
without explanation they inhibit communication and learning. Any 'take
it or leave it' contribution to team effort is likely to increase
demarcation between members, and to inhibit co-operation with a consequent
loss of efficiency. Furthermore it has been shown that complex tasks,
of the sort we are concerned with here, cannot be learnt from outcome
feedback alone (Hammond et al, 1973). The fact that the expert agrees
or disagrees with your judgment does not help you in your next attempt.
The rather subjective decisions to prescribe antibiotics could probably
be made more reliable by identifying the factors which have influenced
these decisions. Experiments to do this have identified a large number
of factors, some of them relating to social and environmental factors
which influence antibiotic prescribing behaviour. This allows other
doctors and non-medical members of the team greater insight into the
otherwise secret process of judgment.   It also allows these judgments
to be made more reliably by the doctor himself. Control may be further
improved by identifying the relative importance of the factors (for
example), thus exposing the principles or rules governing the combination
of data to reach the final judgment. This level of control is similar
to that of the pharmacist monitoring prescription safety. Doctors
and clinical pharmacologists who carry out epidemiological studies or
clinical trials to discover optimal treatments become involved in
judgments which are less and less subjective and increasingly objective.
These decision-making activities of doctors and pharmacists may be
plotted on a continuous scale (Hammond 1978) which for convenience I have
divided into the six categories of which I have just given you
illustrations (Fig.1). They have been classified according to their
mode of cognition whether this is mainly analytical (as in dispensing) or
mainly intuitive (as in the doctor's clinical opinion). Because the
first three activities involve some degree of manipulation and control
over the environment they may be loosely called 'experimental'. The
latter three lack this and are essentially 'judgmental'. I am sure you

have noticed that doctors disagree about decisions involving clinical opinion more often than pharmacists argue about the correct way to fill a prescription.   The difference is that a prescription can be clearly stated and the process of compounding and presenting it is fairly standard. The same cannot be said of many medical decisions where neither the data nor the process of integrating it is explicit.   This does not in any way invalidate decisions reached in this way but it means that disagreements cannot be resolved by an examination of the data and of the process by which data were transmuted into decisions.   The potential for reaching an agreement can be improved by turning to a more analytical mode of thought (more like a pharmacist, you might say) in which the basis for decision is available for discussion.   If this discussion reveals disagreement about what are matters of fact these may then be resolved by a search for more information or by experiment.

If the patient's problems are to be most efficiently tackled by a team approach the members must appreciate and optimise the use of each others skills.   I have tried to show that the practice of medicine and the practice of pharmacy tend to occupy opposite ends of the cognitive

Fig.1 Cognitive activities of doctors and
       pharmacists.

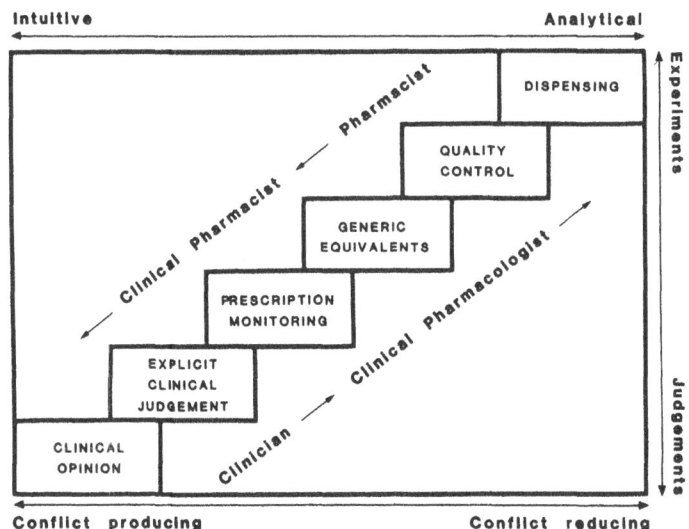

continuum. And it may be that doctors and pharmacists prefer it that way. What is the importance of this observation to the therapeutic team and how does it affect the delivery of patient care?

Firstly, because of the biological environment in which patients' problems occur, control over the circumstances of diagnosis, treatment and follow-up is not possible. Some degree of human judgment will therefore always be needed. Secondly, the exercise of clinical judgment is usually regarded as the doctor's exclusive prerogative. It is often conducted at a subconscious level and its components are therefore hidden from the rest of the team. This prevents them from improving the quality of the decisions by supplying more appropriate information. Studies with rheumatologists have shown that it is possible to reveal the components of clinical judgment. Furthermore, that the information the doctor believes he needs is not what he actually uses. In situations where this information is supplied by other team members clinical judgment analysis could improve the quality of judgments by improving the quality of data on which they are based. Here, for example (Fig.2) are the data which a particular rheumatologist believes he needs to help him judge the effect of treatments on

Fig.2. Measured and perceived contributions of
        clinical variables to judgments.
        (Al = articular index, FC = functional capacity,
        Pain = pain score, EMS = early morning stiffness,
        GLOBAL = patient's overall opinion).

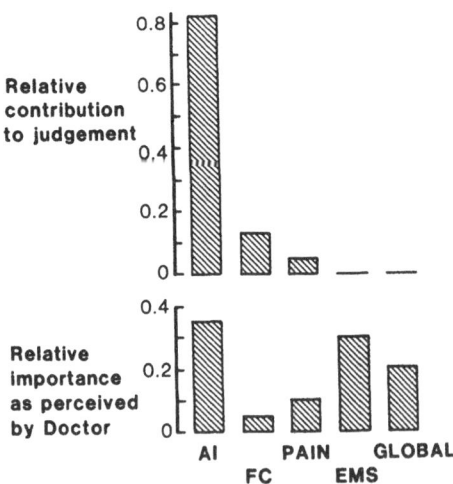

rheumatoid arthritis.   This is the lower set of columns, the height of
each one being proportional to its importance as seen by the doctor.
You will see that some he gets himself, like the number of affected
joints (A1), some the patient gives him, like this global assessment
(GLOBAL), and some might come from an occupational therapist like the
functional capacity (FC). Now look at an objective analysis of the same
doctor's judgment (upper set). He is not actually using the patient's
global assessment at all, but relies mainly on his own view of the
number of affected joints. (Kirwan et al.1983).

Thirdly, as clinical pharmacists approach the biological end
of the cognitive continuum they will find a soft, subjective element
creeping into their data.   The nature of acetyl salicylic acid, for
example, is not something we usually question. But take the question,
"What is an adverse drug reaction?" It may sound easy to define but in
real life even experienced clinicians cannot agree about whether a given
event was really caused by the patient's treatment.   Clinical pharmacists
and nurses are often called upon to make these decisions but I don't
think their judgments will agree any more often than those of doctors.
An adverse drug reaction, on the other hand, while it can be defined in
words, there is little agreement on what actually constitutes one in
practice.   Pharmacists therefore need to be aware that some of the
information they contribute to assist team decisions may involve an
element of judgment and not therefore be of the same quality as the
pharmaceutical data with which they usually work.   Furthermore that
these judgments may be a source of disagreement which can nevertheless
be resolved in the same way as those of their medical colleagues.
Finally, I believe that the concepts of judgment analysis and the cognitive continuum may show what doctors and clinical pharmacists may usefully
learn from each other.   For the doctor, that a better control over
treatment decisions may be achieved by a more precise and scientific
attitude to medical judgment.   For the clinical pharmacist that the amount
of biological variation inherent in most clinical problems makes many of
his solutions over-precise. A greater recognition of the natural
constraints under which most doctors operate seems likely to improve the
relevance of the clinical pharmacist's contribution to the therapeutic
team.

REFERENCES

1.   Hammond, K.R.(1978). Towards increasing competance of thought
            in public policy formation. In Judgment and decision
            in policy formation, ed.K.R.Hammond, pp 11 - 32.
2.   Hammond, K.R., Summers, D.A. and Dean, D.H. (1973). Negative
            effects of outcome feedback in multiple-cue probability
            learning.   Organisational behaviour and human
            performance, 9, 30 - 34.
3.   Kirwan, J.R.,Chaput de Saintonge, D.M., Joyce, C.R.B. & Currey,
            H.L.F (1983). Clinical Judgment in Rheumatoid Arthritis II.
            Judging "Current disease activity" in clinical practice.
            (in press).

THE CONCEPT OF THE THERAPEUTIC TEAM. THE VIEW OF AN ACADEMIC

A.A. Vercruysse
Vrije Universiteit Brussel, Belgium

I think that everyone can agree that the role and the task of of the pharmacist have changed enormously in the last decennia.

Until to-day in the educational programs of our universities the student receive a training in preparing and dispensing medicines. Through their courses of chemistry, physics, biochemistry, statistics, analytical and pharmaceutical chemistry, pharmacognosy and galenics they learn to dispense a medicine of good quality.

Through the courses in anatomy and physiology, pharmacology and toxicology they become able to understand the use, the effects and the toxicity of the therapeutics.

Although the qualification as a dispensing pharmacist (general practice) stays the main objective of the training at academic level, other tasks and functions have emerged. Starting in the fifty's a pharmacist can take functions in the industry (for example as product manager or in the quality control), in hospitals as dispensing and clinical pharmacist, in clinical biology.

For these new qualifications the universities started for each of the new fields a curriculum with courses and practical work. This educational program put on the market technical skilled people.

The question has to be posed if this is the right or the best education and training for pharmacist. We live in a world where health profession have become aware to consider the total patient not just his disease. Besides, the sick person must be placed in his environment.

According to the function of the pharmacist in a dispensing pharmacy, in a hospital, in a laboratory or in an industry, the relationship with the patient is very different.

The dispensing pharmacist (general practice) has the closest relationship with the patient, then comes the hospital pharmacist who dispense his medicines through the nurse. The pharmacist in the industry and the clinical biologist stay still further away from the patient.

Besides the relationship with his patients the dispensing pharmacist as well in the community as in the hospital has a lot of other people and services to communicate with.

In the general practice the pharmacist has to be able to communicate with the prescribers (general practioner, the specialist, the dentist), psychosocial organisations and services (public assistance, centre of family planning, family assistance, infant welfare centre, home care, A.A., etc.), or official services (social security, insurance, justice, health insurance, pension fund, etc.) and other health care services (hospitals, psychiatric institutions, etc.). The hospital pharmacist both in his function as dispensing and as clinical pharmacist lives in a much closer community. The function of a pharmacist in a hospital fits in a health care team and is a part of a therapeutic care team. Not only must he be able to communicate with people of the medical and non-medical staff, but a close cooperation on a more continuous base between some members must exist.

This cooperation results in a therapeutic team with multidisciplinary approach. The people in such a team are :

the medical staff
the nurses
the social nurses and assistants
the clinical biologist
the toxicologist.

The kind of problems that can be treated through this team are :

selection of drugs
optimalisation of therapeutic scheme
drug interaction
drug compliance
automedication
patient counseling and education
cost/benefit analysis.

Further more, the pharmacist has to communicate with :

     the administration and financial service

     the technical services

     the laboratory

     the social service.

In all these instances the pharmacist communicates with people who speak a different language and have their own background and education.

Is the pharmacist prepared for his inclusion in the therapeutic team and in his role as pharmacist in a hospital ? I do not hesitate to answer yes about his technical skill, but he is not prepared and trained for his role in the therapeutic team.

In order to remedy this shortcoming in the education of pharmacist in whatever role they stay in society, we must introduce a course on social science (economic and political sciences) and behavioral sciences (psychology, socio-psychology, sociology). Through this course they should acquire practice in communication and contacts with the patient and interaction with other health professionals and social and health care institutions.

At that moment we should be able to qualify the pharmacist not only for his dispensing role of qualitative and quantitative good drugs but also for optimalisation of the therapy, the quality of care and a concomitant cost containment.

PARENTERAL NUTRITION - THE TEAM APPROACH IN A GENERAL HOSPITAL

M.O. RODRIGUES*, M.E. CAMILO**, M.L. TAVARES**. Departments of Pharmacy* and Medicine II**, University Hospital of Sta. Maria, Lisbon, Portugal.

The present communication is based on the experience of a team in Parenteral Nutrition, who work at a General Hospital with 1 500 beds.

The team is composed mainly of three persons: a clinical pharmacist and two gastroenterology physicians.

We usually follow adult in-patients who need nutritional support either in surgical or medical departments.

MATERIAL AND METHODS

We now present data concerning 70 patients observed from October 1979 to April 1982.

The age of patients ranged from 12 to 75 years. The highest number of patients were between 50 and 70 years.

The patients were divided in three groups: First group - 35 with enterocutaneous fistulas. The main causes of the fistula formation were post-operative or after trauma. The second group - included 27 patients submitted to gastrointestinal surgery: 16 had pre and post-operative nutritional support and 11 had parenteral nutrition only after surgery. Finally the third group - with 8 patients included other clinical situations like intestinal obstruction, pancreatic ascites, which were overcome without surgery.

Our schemes of Parenteral Nutrition were set within caloric values of normonutrition.

The following nutrients were used:

- Glucose in a daily average amount of 297.3 $\pm$ 94.2 grams (mean $\pm$ 1SD). In some patients, we administered Insulin into the bottles of glucose, to prevent hyperglycemia, and at the same time to induce an anabolic effect.

- Lipids were infused in a daily average amount of 31.4 $\pm$ 15.6 grams (mean $\pm$ 1S.D.), through Intralipid emulsion.

In 10/70 (14%) of total patients – with uncontrolled sepsis, pancreatic disease, hyperlipidemia – the only caloric source was glucose.

In the patients with uncontrolled sepsis we observed a delay in clarification of the lipids from the blood. It has been suggested that the relatively slow rate of removal of Intralipid from blood in these patients, may be limited by the amount of carnitine available. This could justify in the future the inclusion of carnitine in parenteral nutrition regimen to enhance the utilization of intravenous lipids.

– Nitrogen was administered in a daily average amount of 9 ± 1.95 grams (mean ± 1SD) through Vamin with glucose.

We supplied a mean of 155.8 ± 29.25 grams (mean±1SD)kilocalories for each gram of nitrogen.

The electrolytes Na,K, HPO_4, Ca and Mg,were normaly administered daily by infusion into the bottles of glucose. The addition was made by the nurses in the ward, with aseptical technique, immediatly before administration to the patients. The electrolytes were used in individual solutions, and we paid attention to possible incompatibilities.

Fig. 1 shows mean values of electrolytes administered in the three groups of patients.

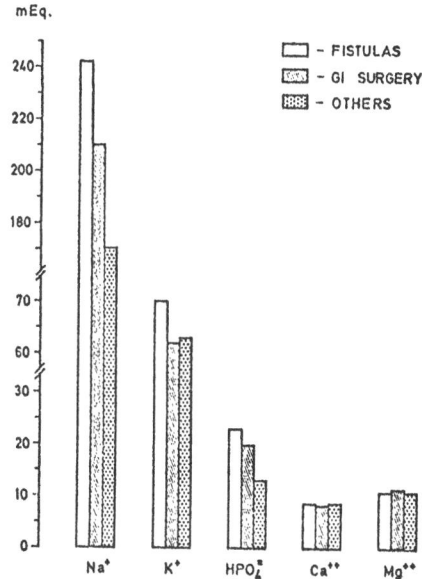

FIG.1 – PARENTERAL NUTRITION: ELECTROLYTES (MEAN/DAY)

Enterocutaneous fistulas needed higher amounts of Na,K and HPO$_4$ than other groups. However the difference was only statistically significant for Na and P when compared with patients without surgery (p $<$ 0.05).

During the scheme of Parenteral Nutrition it is essential to maintain the electrolytes within normal values, in order to attain better metabolism of the nutrients.

The nutrients administration was through a conventional system, over 24 hours. The amino-acid solution was infused concomitantly with glucose or with lipids, through a Y system connected to the intravenous route, either central or peripheral.

The duration of Parenteral Nutrition was from 5 to 50 days. Most of patients had nutritional support between 5 and 20 days.

RESULTS

Besides the general improvement in the clinical situations, an increase of albumin values at the end of Parenteral Nutrition was observed in all groups of patients.

Fig. 2 shows, for example, the significant changes observed before and after in the group of enterocutaneous fistulas.

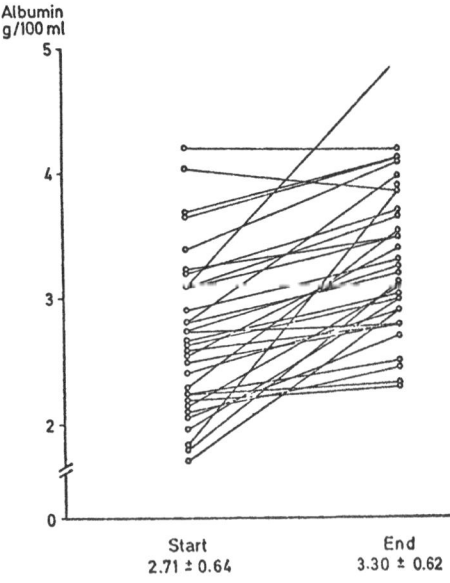

FIG. 2 - ENTEROCUTANEOUS FISTULAS: ALBUMIN VALUES

The main complication observed was catheter fever in about 14% of the patients. The situation was settled by the removal of the intravenous line.

Meanwhile our team has been providing specific education and information to the nurses. Therefore at the present time we have fewer septic complications than when we started.

No significant metabolic complications were registered. A transient small rise in transaminases was observed in 3 patients.

There were 2 allergic reactions to Intralipid and 1 to Vamin, proved by rechallenge.

IN CONCLUSION

Parenteral Nutrition is an important therapy of enterocutaneous fistulas. A spontaneous closure without surgery,was obtained in 71% of them.

It is also a valuable tool in the management of patients undergoing gastrointestinal surgery.

There was usually an improvement in albumin values.

Catheter related fever was the main complication,though without significant morbidity.

The team approach, either directly or by educational programs has lowered risks and improves the efficacy of Parenteral Nutrition.

REFERENCES

Grant, J.P. (1980). Total Parenteral Nutrition. W.B. Saunders Company.

Johnston, I.D.A. (1978). Advances in Parenteral Nutrition, M.T.P. Press Limited.

Kettlewell, M.G.W. (1980). Parenteral Feeding: Practical aspects. Topics in Gastroenterology, ed. S.C. Truelove and H. J. Kennedy, p.p. 33 −42. Blackwell Scientific publications.

Maebashi M., Kawmusa N., Sato M. et al. (1977). Metabolism, 26, 357.

Nehme, A.E. (1980). The Team Concept, JAMA, 243: 1905 − 1908.

Ross, B.D. (1980). Parenteral Feeding: Biochemical considerations. Topics in Gastroenterology, ed. S.C. Truelove and H. J. Kennedy,p.p.15 −31. Blackwell Scientific publications.

LONG-TERM FOLLOW-UP IN TOTAL PARENTERAL NUTRITION.
Benifits of using mixtures in a surgical unit.

Dr.Meersschaut D.,M.D.,Dr.H.Van den Bavière M.D.,

Dr.J.De Roose M.D., Prof.Dr.F.Derom M.D..

Department of Surgery - Academic Hospital Ghent
Belgium.

In 1978, we started using mixtures in total parenteral nutrition (TPN) at the Academic hospital in Gent.
Up to then, starting in 1972, TPN was administered under the form of separated, commercially available, solutions. To facilitate the administration of mixtures, they were standardised in 8 types and later in 4 types depending on the patients need for calories and nitrogen.
The original solutions ranged from 900 Kcal and 7,6 grN up to 3200 Kcal and 18grN. All solutions respected the generally accepted Kcal/grN ratio of about 150. The solutions were adopted for experimental reasons in 1980. For the year 1981 the number of mixtures was reduced to 4 : the steps between the upgrading solutions were considered as too small and the mixing process became much easier   with a smaller number of solutions.
At the moment we use 4 solutions from 1250 Kcal and 7,6 grN up to 16,8 grN and 2500 Kcal.
Trace-elements were added to the solutions starting from the third week of administration.
Lipids, commercially available as Intralipid, were used in concentrations of 10 and 20 per cent.
They represent 40 per cent of the total calorie demand.

To check the benifits of mixtures we did compare them with the classical separated TPN.

Cathetersepsis and the possibility to stop anastomatic leaks by TPN alone were choosen as parameters for ease of use and clinical effectiveness.

Our population consists of 562 patients, of which 158 received mixtures. They were all operated for gastro-intestinal anastomatics. They were checked for age, sex, type of operation, cathetersepsis, frequency of anastomatic leaks and duration of parenteral nutrition. In total 158 patients received 1886 days TPN-mixtures, this means an average period of 12 days parenteral nutrition.(Table 1).

All TPN was administrated by central venous catheter because of hyperosmolarity of the used fluids.

In discussing cathetersepsis we must distinguish 3 exogenous factors : - sterility of mixtures,

- contamination of connections,

- sterility of puncture and puncture-site.

Table 1   PATIENTS SUBMITTED TO TPN

	nr.of pt.	nr.of days	Max.	Min.	Mean
78 :	9 (58)	85	18	8	9,43
79 :	43 (51)	512	37	6	12,03
80 :	40 (50)	531	40	6	14,15
81 :	66 (75)	758	34	4	11,53

Mixtures were made under laminar air-flow respecting absolute
sterile conditions, everything was   mixed   by hand. During the
3 years, checking for contamination revealed no positive result.
For large scale application of TPN, this method was too comple-
cated so we develloped a method of mixing and filling up large
numbers of bags at a time. Mixing   is done under non-sterile
conditions, and filtrated afterwards for particles, pyrogenous
substances and bacteria. All connections are sanitary-fittings
and bags are filled under laminar   air-flow, lipids are added.
The fimal solution is stable for more than 24 hours at room-
temperature , this is the time needed for administration. E.V.A.-
bags are used to prevent destabilsation of lipid-suspensions.

Contamination of the connections is closely related
to the number of connections in the system. In the classical
system patient was connected to some kind of X-mas-tree, with
many connectins, which means, for long term TPN, simply asking
for cathetersepsis. Up to now for the last 3 years we use for
TPN only one side-line for administration of lipids, both lines
being changed withe the bags   every 24 hours. The new "all-in
one-bag" will make side-lines completely obsolete.
Adding medication to the bags is forbidden to avoid contamination.

Sterility of puncture-site, the third factor of cathetersepsis, is at the moment the most difficult to handle.
But the introduction of a specialized nurse, handling only ca-
theter-dressings, seems to be an important improvement.
Table 2 shows two clear, statistically significant drops in ca-
thetersepsis-rate.(Calculated on 100 days of TPN). The first
corresponds with the introductions of mixtures, the second

with the new scheme of catheter-care.

The second part of the studies deals withe the healing of anastomatic leaks. The frequency af   anastomatic _leaks
depends on the localisation of the anastomosis, on the
surgical technique and on the nutritional status of the patient.
Therefore only healing of an existing leak was accepted as a
parameter of effectiveness of the parenteral nutrition. All
patients suffering from anastomatic leaks were treated with TPN.
Surgical reintervention was only perform if intestinal situation of the patient remained difficult to handle with parenta-
ral nutrition. Oral feeding was started after X-ray-control.
The number of cured leaks was considered as an indication that
we supplied enough nitrogen in a well balanced calorie/Nitro-
gen proportion to simulate anabolism   enough to heal the de-
fect in the intestinal wall.

Table 2

NUMBER OF ISOLATED CATHETERSEPSIS ON
CENTRAL INFUSION-LINES.

	n	d C.I.	n/100 d. C.I.
72	8	150	5,3
73	6	124	4,8
74	9	210	4,2
75	10	264	3,8
76	13	351	3,7
77	23	510	4,5
78	10	348 (85)	2,8 (2,3)
79	10	512	1,9
80	10	531	1,9
81	7	758	0,9

The number of the cured leaks dropped sigificantly after introduction of mixtures (table 3). This is in our opnion, a
clear advantage of mixtures compared with the seaprate solutions.

As a conclusion we can say that :

1. The use of mixtures in parenteral nutrition lowers the frequency of cathetersepsis. This means safer nutrition with both
lower morbidity and mortality. This also allows administration
without interruptions, making the alimentation more effective.

2. A higher and better balanced Nitrogen and calorie supply
makes leaks heal better and decreases the necessity of surgical reIntervention.

Table 3   NUMBER OF   ANASTOMATIC   LEAKS

pt.	leaks	%	cured leaks by TPN	%
72	51	9	17,6	5	55
73	57	12	21,0	6	50
74	46	10	21,7	6	60
75	53	10	18,9	5	50
76	54	12	22	4	33
77	62	8	12,9	4	50
78	58	9 (3) 15,5	4 (3)	33 (100)
79	51	10	19,6	8	80
80	50	8	16	6	75
81	75	12	16	9	75

TOTAL PARENTERAL NUTRITION OF CHILDREN AT THE STATE UNIVERSITY
HOSPITAL OF COPENHAGEN

M. Rasmussen
Royal Danish School of Pharmacy, DK-2100 Copenhagen, Denmark

K. Nordfjeld
Royal Danish School of Pharmacy, DK-2100 Copenhagen, Denmark

P.V. Pedersen
Frederiksborg County Hospital, DK-2970 Hørsholm, Denmark

Abstract. Total parenteral nutrition of children demands a
close cooperation between all professionals involved in the
therapy. Nutrition of a 6-year-old boy is used to illustrate
the influence of several factors on the therapy. The boy has
received total parenteral nutrition (TPN) for 40 months because the absorption of nutrients from the gastrointestinal
tract was insufficient. Parenteral nutrition with amino acids,
lipids, carbohydrates, electrolytes, and vitamins has - until
his death in October 1981 - established normal development
physically as well as psychically. Introduction of parenteral
nutrition mixtures prepared centrally at the hospital pharmacy
drastically reduced both the incidence of septic episodes and
the use of antibiotics in comparison with traditional preparation of the mixture on the ward.

INTRODUCTION

Traditionally hospital pharmacies in Denmark produce simple
parenteral solutions used in the hospitals on a large scale, e.g. glucose
and electrolyte solutions. In addition the hospital pharmacies often produce some solutions of more complex character for specific groups of patients - solutions produced in large batches and stored after heat treatment. This kind of preparation is not staff consuming compared with patient specific preparation including additive service, for which the staff
capacity in Danish hospital pharmacies is insufficient (Table 1).

The State University Hospital of Copenhagen has about 2,000
beds. The sterile production includes all forms of preparations - infusions in glass bottles, infusions in plastic bags, vials, ampoules, hemo-
dialyses, peritonealdialyses, eyedrops, ointments - and amounts to a total of 3/4 million units per year. Aseptic preparations amount only to
about 6,000 units per year.

Normally when patients are fed parenterally the hospital
pharmacy delivers the standard solutions, and all admixtures of additives
are performed by the nurse on the ward. In a very few instances the ste-

rile department of the pharmacy has prepared all solutions to a specific patient including all additives and made them ready to use. The paper will describe such a case.

CASE HISTORY

With the diagnosis of pseudo-Hirschsprung's disease a boy has received TPN from the age of 2½ years till 6 when he died. A variety of diagnostic tests and a few operative solutions have been applied without establishing a sufficient absorptive capacity in the intestinal tract.

TPN with amino acids, lipids, carbohydrates, electrolytes, trace elements, and vitamins established normal development psychically as well as physically.

Within the TPN period the boy had 54 surgical venous exposures mostly on account of septicemia.

In 1980 the procedures for preparation of the TPN solutions were changed to reduce, if possible, the frequences of periods of septicemia.

Further information on this case is published in Progress in Clinical Pharmacy III, 1981 (2).

MATERIALS AND METHODS

TPN-solutions

During the first 2 years of the treatment the solutions were made ready for use by the nurses on the ward as described below under period 1.

Table 1. Staff at the State University Hospital Pharmacy

	Hospital pharmacy	
	Dept. of sterile prod.	Total
Pharmacists	1	11
Technicians	4	22
Unskilled personnel	13	31
Total	18	64

During the remaining period solutions were made ready for use in the aseptic department in the hospital pharmacy as described below under period 2.

Period 1: Preparation method

The nurses obtained amino acids and lipids from the hospital pharmacy in the form of Vamin Comp. RH and Intralip 20%, which were administered without additives. Vamin Comp. RH is specially composed for children. The mixture of amino acids, carbohydrates, and electrolytes is prepared in batches in the hospital pharmacy and finished with a heat treatment for 20 minutes at 80 °C. The composition of the mixture is shown in Table 2.

Table 2.   Composition of Vamin Comp. RH

Amino acids g/l

Isoleucine	1.3	Total nitrogen g/l	3.1
Leucine	1.8	Carbohydrates g/l	
Lysine	1.3		
Phenylalanine	1.8	Fructose	33.3
Methionine	0.6	Glucose	60.7
Threonine	1.0		
Tryptophan	0.3	Energy per l (kJ)	1900
Valine	1.4	Electrolytes mmol/l	
Essential amino acids	9.6	Sodium	16.7
		Potassium	19.0
Cysteic acid/Cystine	0.5	Calcium	0.83
Tyrosine	0.2	Magnesium	2.1
Alanine	1.0	Acetate	–
Arginine	1.1	Chloride	18.3
Aspartic acid	1.4	Sulphate	2.1
Glutamine acid	3.0	Phosphate	12.3
Glycine	0.7	Lactate	–
Histidine	0.8		
Proline	2.7	Osmolarity mOsm/l	780
Serine	2.5	pH	5
Non-essential amino acids	13.8		
Total amino acids	23.4		

Carbohydrates and electrolytes were delivered as an autoclaved solution produced in batches by the hospital pharmacy. The product is called Invertose-Darrow (Table 3). Within one day the patient had 3 bottles of 350 ml for administration in the following way:

1st bottle: 100 ml were removed and disposed of. To the remaining 250 ml were added:

    40   ml Ped-el from 2 vials (electrolytes and trace elements)

    0.5   ml Pancebrin from 1 vial (vitamins)

    1.0   ml Phytomenadione from 2 ampoules (= 0.5 mg)

    0.25 ml Folic Acid from 1 ampoule (= 2.5 mg)

    35   ml Sodium Chloride from 1 vial (= 35 mmol)

    8   ml Potassium Chloride from 1 vial (= 8 mmol)

    20   ml Magnesium Chloride from 1 vial (10 mmol)

2nd bottle: 100 ml were removed and disposed of. To the remaining 250 ml were added:

    35   ml Ped-el from 2 vials

    35   ml Sodium Chloride from 1 vial

    10   ml Potassium Chloride from 1 vial

    5   ml Potassium Phosphate from 1 vial (= 5 mmol)

Table 3. Composition of Invertose-Darrow (Liquor Darrow, Inf. invertose 100 g/l   1+3)

Carbohydrates	7.5 %
Glucose	37.5 g/l
Fructose	37.5 g/l
Energy	1190 kJ/l
Electrolytes	
Sodium	31 mmol/l
Potassium	9
Chloride	26
Lactate	14
pH	5.1
Osmolarity	500 mOsm/l

3rd bottle: 100 ml were removed and disposed of. To the remaining 250 ml
    were added:

    30 ml Sodium Chloride from 1 vial

    8 ml Potassium Chloride from 1 vial

Period 2: Preparation method

The preparation in the hospital pharmacy took place in the
aseptic department in a laminar air flow bench and the personnel were
dressed for aseptic procedures. The normal pharmaceutical practice including preparation of master chart, pharmaceutical supervision of the
technicians, etc. was observed. The following 5 bottles were prepared
every day and delivered to the ward ready to use.

    to Vamin Comp. RH 450 ml were added 80 ml (4x20 vials) Ped-el

    to Invertose-Darrow 1000 ml were added 5 ml Soluvit from 1 vial

    to Invertose-Darrow 500 ml were added 3 ml Soluvit from 1 vial

    to Intralipid 20% 85 ml were added 8 ml Vitalipid from 1 vial

    to Intralipid 20% 85 ml were added 8 ml Vitalipid from 1 vial

The daily administration of nutrients is listed in Table 4.

Table 4. Daily nutrition

Volume (123 ml/kg)	1845	ml	Carbohydrates	600	cals
Amino acids	10,5	g	Fat	300	cals
Na^+	105	mEq	Cl^-	125	mEq
K^+	27	mEq	$Phosphate^-$	7,25	mEq
Ca^{++}	41	mEq	$Lactate^-$	6,6	mEq
Mg^{++}	29	mEq	I^-	0,5	µEq
Fe^{+++}	187	µEq	F^-	37,5	µEq
Mn^{++}	25	µEq			
Zn^{++}	15	µEq			
Cu^{++}	15	µEq			
Ascorbic acid	15	mg	Folate	2	mg
Thiamine	2,5	mg	Vitamin A	2500	IU
Riboflavin	0,5	mg	Vitamin D	250	IU
Niacin	50	mg	Vitamin E	0,5	mg
Pantothenic acid	0,75	mg	Vitamin K	0,5	mg
Pyridoxine	0,75	mg	Vitamin B_{12} monthly	1	mg

Clinical evaluation

All data on the numbers of bacteriologically verified inci-
dences of septicemia and the administration of antibiotics are collected
retrospectively from the medical record.

RESULTS AND DISCUSSION

The patient received TPN for a total of 40 months of his 6
years of life. Within the first 23 months the preparation of the TPN solutions took place at the ward in a non-sterile environment as previously
described under period 1. During this period the boy was hospitalized continuously except for visits of a few hours at home. He went through 17
periods of septicemia demanding removal of the central catheter followed
by surgical replacement of the catheter in anaesthesia. As it takes some
days to test whether a fever is caused by infection in the blood, it is
necessary to start an antibiotic treatment at once without knowing the
cause of the fever. For this reason the boy was heavily treated with antibiotics as shown in Table 5.

Table 5. Episodes of septicemia and use of antibiotics

	period 1*	period 2**
Numbers of septicemic episodes	17	3
Numbers of periods with use of antibiotics		
Ampicillin	12	4
Benzylpenicillin	0	1
Carbenicillin	0	1
Cephalothin	1	0
Gentamicin	24	3
Meticillin	17	1
Sulphamathoxazole, Trimethoprim	1	1
Total	55	11

* Period 1: April 1978 to May 1980 with preparation at the ward.

** Period 2: June 1980 to October 1981 with aseptical preparation
              at the hospital pharmacy

When the boy was 4½ years of age the hospital pharmacy took over the preparation of the TPN mixtures and thereby made it possible for his parents to handle the administration. During the following 17 months the boy often stayed at home, where he played in the daytime as other kids and was fed parenterally over night while asleep. During this period of time he had only two incidents of septicemia (Table 5). The reduced incidence of septicemia might be a result of several things of which aseptic preparation of the TPN solutions could be one and the removal of the boy from the hospital environment another. It has previously been reported that TPN treatment at home gives a lower indicence of sepsis (I).

However, the patient died when 6 years old from a septicemia caused by candida and moreover, at that time no further venous access for parenteral nutrition was available. The patient had then had 54 venous exposures.

CONCLUSION

It has been possible to improve the life quality during more than a year for one patient by changing some hospital routines in Denmark. A general conclusion cannot be made from this single case as to whether the preparation method in period 2 is better than the preparation method in period 1 because many factors influence the incidence of septicemia.

However this case illustrates the complexity of treatment of TPN children. TPN treatment should be planned and taken care of by a team with special training and knowledge about TPN treatment. The team should at any time have the responsibility of the treatment. In this context, the nurse on duty would be able to rely on comprehensive recommendations. The team members could be a physician and/or a surgeon, a nurse, and a pharmacist, and in addition it would be of great help to have consultants attached to the team, e.g. a psychiatrist and a dietician. In the treatment of TPN children it is of great importance to involve the parents in the child's therapy. Most parents are willing and able to handle the administration of TPN solutions at home, and even if it is not possible to prove a diminished risk of septicemia yet, the improvement of the patient's life quality is obvious.

References

Ladefoged, K., Efsen, F., Christoffersen, J. Krogh & Jarnum, S. (1981).
Long-term parenteral nutrition. II. Catheter-related complications. Scand. J. Gastroenterology, 16 (7) p. 913-919.

Pedersen, P.V. (1981). 4½-year-old boy on parenteral nutrition for 2 years. Progress in Clinical Pharmacy III, ed. H. Turakka and E. van der Kleijn, p.277-80. Elsevier, Holland.

COMPATIBILITY OF TWO DIFFERENT FAT EMULSIONS WITH AMINOACIDS, CARBOHYDRATES AND ELECTROLYTES IN PARENTERAL NUTRITION MIXTURES

H. Pamperl
I[st] University Clinic of Gastroenterology and Hepatology, School of Medicine, University of Vienna, Austria

G. Kleinberger
I[st] University Clinic of Internal Medicine, School of Medicine, University of Vienna, Austria

Abstract. The ultrastructure of an egg lecithin (Intralipid[R] 20%) and a soya phosphatide (Lipofundin[R]-S 20%) stabilized fat emulsion was investigated by a transmission electron microscope before and after the contact with the other components of so called "All in one" (AIO)-solutions. In the native egg lecithin stabilized emulsion the particles appeared homogeneous, sometimes carrying inclusion bodies. Soya phosphatide stabilized fat droplets appeared homogeneous too, but the electron density of the surface rim was weaker, the number of inclusion bodies was higher. Highly concentrated carbohydrates provoked a rapid deterioration of both emulsion systems. Addition of aminoacids produced numerous inclusion bodies but no coalescence or confluence. Electrolytes in amounts used in AIO-solutions had no effect on the lipid particles ultrastructure. Mixing all the components of AIO-solutions together with adding the fat emulsions as the last step produced no further alterations in the fat particles as seen after the contact with aminoacids alone in particular the carbohydrate related effect was avoided.

Key words: fat emulsions, intravenous - parenteral feeding - compatibility - electron microscopy.

INTRODUCTION

In a previous study (Pamperl & Kleinberger 1982) we could show that the contact of an egg lecithin stabilized fat emulsion with the other components necessary for total parenteral nutrition (TPN) provoked the formation of inclusion bodies within the fat droplets. As mixing of "All In One" (AIO)-solutions for TPN is still not generally accepted we tried to evaluate the effects of the single components of AIO-solutions on the ultrastructure of two different commercially available fat emulsions.

MATERIALS AND METHODS

An egg lecithin (Intralipid[R] 20%) and a soya phosphatide (Lipofundin[R]-S 20%) stabilized fat emulsion were either solely mixed with the single components of AIO-solutions as glucose 30% or 60% (glucose:fat=1:1), Amino-Mel[R] optimal 10% (aminoacids:fat=2:1), electrolytes: sodium 20 mval or 80 mval (as malate) or potassium 40 mval or 80 mval/l (as chloride) or with a 2:1 mixture of aminoacids and glucose 60% or thirdly with all the other components of TPN solution "normal" as described elsewhere (Kleinberger et al. 1981). From the mixtures samples for electron microscopy and pH measurement were taken immediately after preparation and 24 hours later. The pH determinations were carried out by a combined glass electrode type GK 2303 C: Radiometer, Copenhagen, Denmark. Calibrations were done with standard buffer solutions from the electrode producer (buffer S 1326 for pH 7.00 and S 1316 for pH 4.01). After each measurement a cleaning of the electrode by fresh ethanol 70% was undertaken.

Preparation of the specimens for electron microscopy was done as described in detail elsewhere (Pamperl & Kleinberger 1982).A sample of fresh native egg lecithin stabilized emulsion additionally embedded at the 24 hours stage, served as a control.

RESULTS

A) Native fat emulsions:

In the electron microscope the lipid particles of native egg lecithin stabilized fat emulsion were of spherical shape with a slightly

Fig.1 Intralipid[R] 20%, native   Fig.2 Lipofundin[R]-S 20%, native

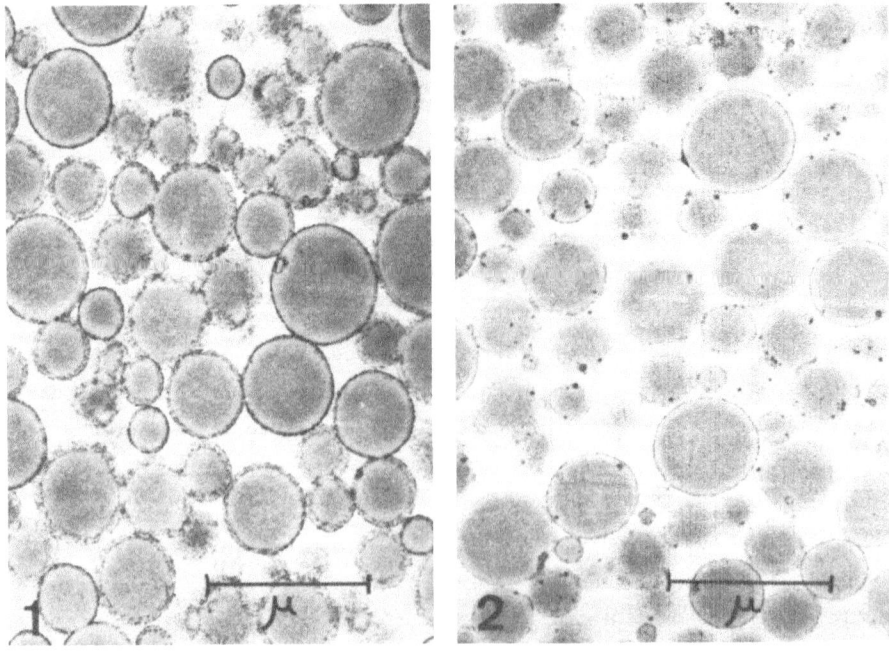

Fig.3 Intralipid[R] 20%, glucose 30% Fig.4 Intralipid[R] 20%, potassium
fresh   80 mval dm^{-3} fresh

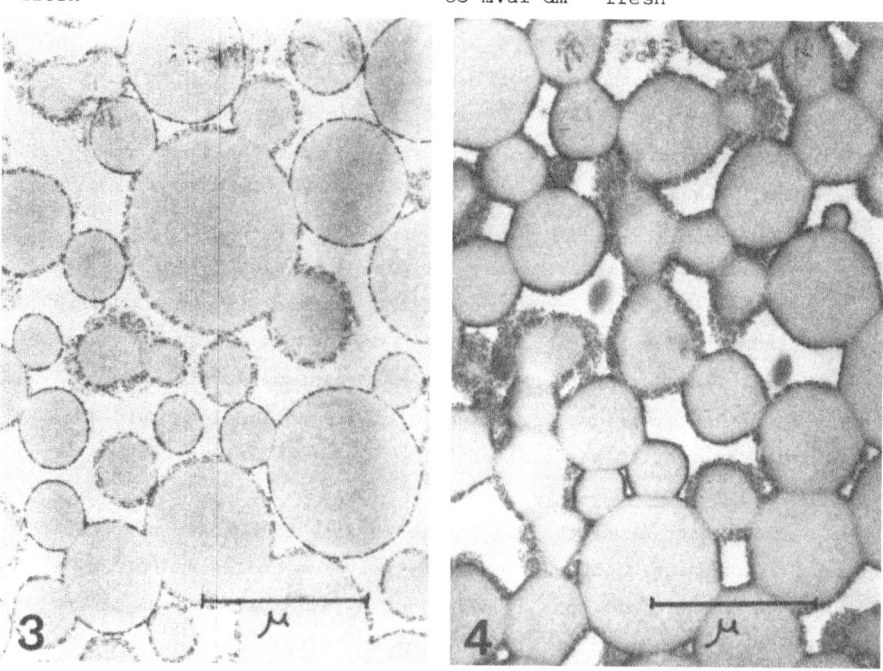

Fig.5 AIO-solution/Intralipid[R] 20% Fig.6 AIO-solution/Lipofundin[R]
fresh   -S 20%, fresh

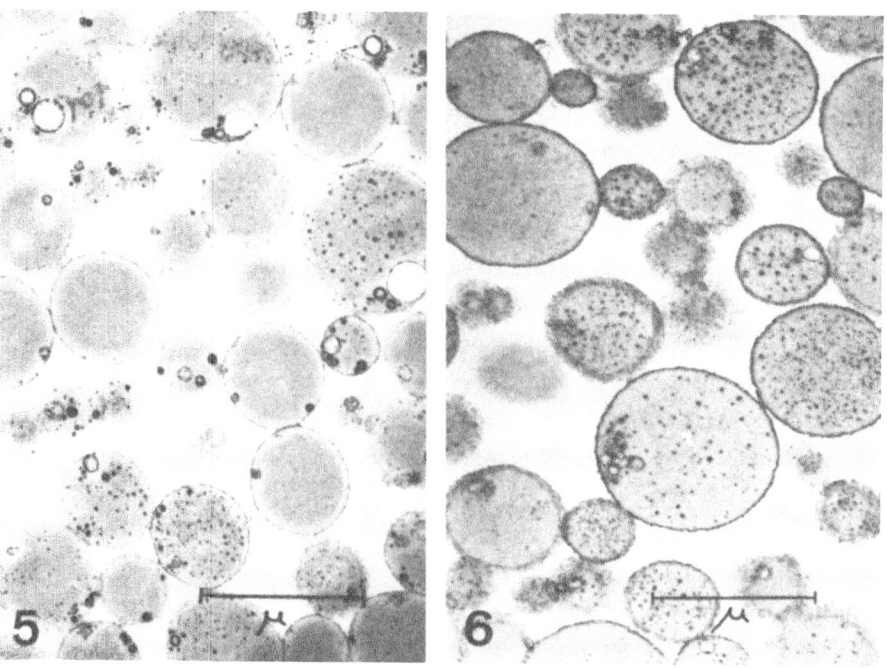

osmiophilic homogeneous center and a highly osmiophilic coarse rim. Sometimes little inclusion bodies were to be seen. Some of the droplets were
attached but no coalescence or confluation was detectable (Fig.1). Fat
particles of soya phosphatide stabilized emulsions were different insofar
as the osmiophility of the surface rim was much weaker and the number of
inclusion bodies was higher (Fig. 2).

B) Carbohydrates:

Immediately after mixing fat emulsions with 60% or 30% glucose
the fat droplets showed interruptions of the surface rim. At the sites of
droplet attachment the limiting borderline diminuated and confluation followed (Fig.3). Giant droplets of more than 30 micrometer could be observed.
After 24 hours the emulsions were floculated and no samples could be embedded. This observation was similar for both fat emulsions tested.

C) Aminoacids:

The contact of the fat particles with aminoacids provoked the
formation of numerous highly osmiophilic inclusion bodies and globules,
but the droplets were not equally affected. A few remained free of inclusion bodies, others beared little vacuoles and others carried only inclusion bodies with a more disperse or a more patchy appearence. These observations were similar in both freshly admixed fat emulsions and no further
change in morphology was detectable 24 hours later. When carbohydrates
were mixed with aminoacids and then added to the fat emulsions the ultrastructure was the same as described for the contact with aminoacids alone.
No further change in ultrastructure was seen after 24 hours.

D) Electrolytes:

Adding of small amounts of monovalent cations as 40 mval sodium or 40 mval potassium had no effect on the fat droplets ultrastructure.
Higher concentrations as 80 mval led to interruptions in the surface rim
and to enhanced attachment of droplets with regard to sodium. Potassium
changed the ultrastructure insofar as nearly all droplets were attached,
presenting a multiangular shape. Between the attached droplets a thin borderline was still present. The free interface of the droplets was thicker
as in the native emulsions (Fig.4).

E) Complete AIO-solutions:

After mixing all the components necessary for TPN together only the alterations seen after the contact with aminoacids alone were observable. Even after 24 hours no further signs of instability as enhanced
attachment or interruption of surface rim occured in both fat emulsions
used (Fig. 5, Fig. 6).

F) pH measurement:

For the results of pH measurements see table 1. It was noted that fat emulsions increased the low pH of highly concentrated carbohydrates from 3.14 to 3.4 and decreased the pH of the aminoacid solution about 0.3. The small amount of added electrolytes had no effect on the fat emulsions pH.

Table 1 pH values of the single components and mixtures of AIO-solutions (n.d.=not done)

	pH				
COMPONENTS		Intralipid[R] 2o%		Lipofundin[R]-S 2o%	
		fresh	24 hours	fresh	24 hours
fat		7.56		6.9o	
Glucose 6o%	3.14	3.45	3.33	3.43	3.25
Glucose 3o%	4.21	4.61	3.91	4.47	3.37
Aminoacids	7.42	7.16	7.13	7.18	7.16
Glucose 6o% and Aminoacids	7.2o	7.o1	7.o4	7.o6	7.o3
Sodium 4o mval	n.d.	7.55	n.d.	6.9o	n.d.
Sodium 8o mval	n.d.	7.51	n.d.	6.89	n.d.
Potassium 4o mval	n.d.	7.58	n.d.	6.9o	n.d.
Potassium 8o mval	n.d.	7.58	n.d.	6.92	n.d.
All components of AIO-solutions	7.o3	6.81	6.8o	6.85	6.87

DISCUSSION

The ultrastructural differences between native egg lecithin and soya phosphatide stabilized emulsions mainly concerned the osmiophility of the fat particles surface rim and their number of inclusion bodies.This is due to the different chemical composition of the emulgators. As osmium is bound to double bonds (Korn 1966 a,b) it is indicated that soya phosphatides have a lower amount of those highly reactive binding sites, although the exact chemical reactions of osmium tetroxide with lipids are still not fully understood (Pearse 1980). Highly concentrated carbohydrates destroyed both emulsifying systems within 24 hours. Even after a few minutes deleterious effects were demonstrable in the electron microscope. This is in accordance with the results of Black and Popovics (1981) who reported about a significant change of particle size distribution after the contact of Intralipid[R] with carbohydrates exceeding 5%. It is likely that this phenomenon is caused by the very low pH (3.14) of carbohydrate solutions which is chosen by the producer to avoid chemical alterations during autoclavation. That lowering of pH itself can provoke phase separation of fat emulsions was firstly reported by Zeringue et al. (1964) for egg lecithin and explained by Shah and Schulman (1967) who mentioned that the phosphatidyl group of the lecithin molecule is neutralized and therefore reversal of the zeta potential becomes possible. This was later on proved by Dawes and Groves (1977). Contact of aminoacids led to the formation of numerous inclusion bodies and globules within the fat droplets of both fat emulsions tested. Still we have no definite explanation for this. Probably it might be an effect of certain aminoacids or of any additive in the solutions necessary for production. It is of great interest that no signs of instability were observable within a period of 24 hours regardless to the emulgator. Complete AIO-solutions are presenting a similar ultrastructure and remain morphologically stable for more than one week as previously reported (Pamperl & Kleinberger 1982). When aminoacids and carbohydrates are mixed together and then added to fat emulsions the carbohydrate related effect can be prevented as the low pH of the carbohydrates is buffered by the aminoacid solutions. Therefore our results morphologically sustain the findings of Black and Popovics (1981). Martin (1941) and Van den Temple (1953) were the first who reported about the incompatibilities of electrolytes with fat emulsions. Dawes and Groves (1978) reported about the discharge of the negative zeta potential of Intralipid liposomes by various electrolytes. Sodium and potassium were found to diminuate the negative charge from -30 mV to - 20 mV when added in amounts of 50 mval. 80 mval discharged further on to -10 mV. This is in good accordance with our findings that agglomeration of droplets is provoked when adding 80 mval to the emulsions. We could observe this in both fat emulsions although Gray and Singleton (1967) had reported that crude phosphatides are stronger stabilizers against electrolytes than pure lecithin. Therefore either electrolyte should not exeed 40 mval when admixed to fat emulsions. This is of great importance insofar as various aminoacid solutions contain different amounts of electrolytes. This should be always kept in mind when mixing AIO-solutions.

In conclusion we found that native Intralipid[R] and Lipofundin[R] revealed some differences with regard to their ultrastructure but no differences in their behaviour against the other components of AIO-solutions. For clinical use we recommend that the fatty components of AIO-solutions as artificial fat emulsions and lipid soluble vitamins should be added as the last step to avoid the carbohydrate effect.

REFERENCES

Black, C.D. & Popovics, N.G. (1981). Drug.Intell.Clin.Pharm.,15, 184-193.
Dawes, W.H. & Groves, M.J. (1978). Int.J.Pharm.,1, 141-150.

Gray, M.S. & Singleton, W.S. (1967). J.Pharm.Sciences,56, 1429-1431.
Kleinberger, G., Druml, W., Grabner, A., Lochs, H. & Pichler, M. (1981).
      Der Krankenhausarzt,54, 23-32.
Korn, E.D. (1966 a). Biochem.Bioph.Acta,116, 317-324.
Korn, E.D. (1966 b). Biochem.Bioph.Acta,116, 325-335.
Martin, A.R. & Hermann, R.N. (1941).Trans.Faraday Soc. 37/3o
Pamperl, H. & Kleinberger, G. (1982). Infusionstherapie,9, 86-91.
Pearse, A.G.E. (1980) Histochemistry,Vol.1, Chapt.5, 114-119
Shah, D.O. & Schulman, J.H. (1967). J.Lipid Res.,8, 227-233.
Van den Temple, M. (1953). Rec.Trav.Chim.,72, 442.
Zeringue, H., Brown, J. & Singleton, W.S. (1964). J.Am.Oil Chem.,41,688-
      691.

ESOPHAGUS CANCER AND PARENTERAL NUTRITION:POSTOPERATIVE
COMPLICATIONS AND P.N.I. RELATIONSHIP.PRELIMINARY STUDY.

Cardona,D.[1];Bassons,T.[1];Sanchez Segura,J.M.[2];Castro I.[1]
and Bonal,J.[1].
Hospital de la Santa Creu i Sant Pau.Barcelona.Spain.
1 Pharmacy Service
2 I.C.U.

Esophagus cancer is not a very frequent problem but
important due to high mortality.

In 1970, in our country this mortality was
5/100.000 men and 1.7/100.000 women.(Prieto,L.1976).

The mean survival rate at five years is 3% (Moertel
C.G.1973;Appelquist,P.1972), dying the majority of patients
during the first or second year after the diagnosis is made.

Several factors can contribute to this low survival
rate as patient age, toxic habits (alcohol,tobacco), too
late diagnosis etc...

The treatment is preoperative radiotherapy and
surgery through total esophaguectomy, gastric interposition
and jejunostomy. The surgical procedure can be made by
thoracotomy according to Torek and Nakayama (1967) or by
stripping according to Akiyama (1980), Ong (1971) and
Mc Keown (1981).

Postoperative mortality has decreased during last
years because of advances in surgery, anesthesia, pre and
postoperative care and parenteral nutrition. However,several
factors remain associated with this high mortality. (See
Table 1).

The purpose of this paper is to check the incidence
of patient nutritional status in the postoperative morbidity
and/or mortality.

For this reason, when patients arrive to the
hospital we studied their nutritional status calculating the
Prognostic Nutritional Index (P.N.I.) according to Mullen
et al.(1980) and we tried to find in a retrospective study

TABLE 1: RISK FACTORS
   1. Patient mean age.
   2. Late diagnosis .Tumors⟩10cm length and nodes invasion.
   3. High risk surgery.
   4. Undernourished patients: Dysphagia
   5. Protein-Calorie malnutrition.

a relationship between P.N.I. and postoperative
complications.

MATERIAL AND METHODS

Ten patients with carcinoma of esophagus were
studied between January-June 1982. These patients
accomplished the inclusion criteria of the oncologic-
surgical protocol established in our hospital.

The age of patients was between 45 and 67 with a
mean age of 54±7.80% of patients were men and 20% were women.

The criteria to exclude patients from the protocol
(Table 2) are the following: besides patients with a
preoperative tumor stage superior to $T_2N_0M_0$, we exclude
patients older than 70 years, with associated cardiopathy
and/or respiratory problems, diabetes, chronic hepatopathy,
renal failure and patients with a weight loss higher than
20% of their usual body weight.

Those patients with body weight loss higher than
20% but that could be recovered with parenteral or enteral
nutrition are included in the protocol.

Patients distribution according to tumor site and
tumor histology is shown in Tables 3 and 4.

The treatment was preoperative radiotherapy with
Co^{60}: 2.000-3.000 rads/T during 4 or 5 days and surgery.
In eight patients surgery was esophaguectomy plus
gastroplasty and jejunostomy. Among these patients the
surgical procedure was thoracotomy in 6 patients and
stripping in 2 patients depending on tumor site. The two
patients left   underwent laparotomy (Table 5).

We assessed the patients nutritional status when

TABLE 2: PATIENT EXCLUDED FROM THE PROTOCOL
1. Tumors stage $>$ to $T_2 N_0 M_0$
2. $>$ 70 years old.
3. Associated cardiopathy and/or respiratory problems
4. Diabetes, Hepatopathy and renal failure.
5. ↓ 20% of usual weight, except patients that can be recovered with parenteral and/or enteral nutrition.

TABLE 3: PATIENTS DISTRIBUTION ACCORDING TO TUMOR SITE

1. Cervical esophagus		0
2. Intrathoracic esophagus	Upper Portion	1
	Middle Portion	4
3. Distal esophagus		5

TABLE 4: PATIENT DISTRIBUTION ACCORDING TO TUMOR HISTOLOGY

1. Squamous cell carcinoma	9
2. Adenocarcinoma	1

TABLE 5: PATIENTS DISTRIBUTION ACCORDING TO TYPE OF OPERATION

Esophaguectomy + gastroplasty +	Stripping	2
Jejunostomy	Thoracotomy	6
Laparotomy		2

they arrive to the hospital according to Blackburn et al. (1977), this study is based in the following parameters: (Tables 6.1 and 6.2).

    1. Anthropometrics:

Standard values of height, weight, triceps skinfold relation between weight loss and time, arm circumference, arm muscle circumference etc. We used our population standard values according to Alastrué et al.(1982).

    2. Laboratory:

Besides visceral proteins with different half life as serum albumin and serum transferrin, cholesterol and creatinine/height index are included.

    3. Immunologic Response:

Total lymphocyte count and skin test antigens

TABLE 6.1: NUTRITIONAL STATUS ASSESSMENT
   1. Anthropometric parameters
      Height   (mts)
      Ideal body weight, usual wt, real wt   (Kg)
      Relation weight loss with time   (Kg)
      Triceps Skinfold   (mm)
      Arm Circumference   (cm)
      Arm muscle circumference   (cm)

TABLE 6.2: NUTRITIONAL STATUS ASSESSMENT
   2. Laboratory parameters
      Creatinine height index
      Serum albumin   gr/1
      Serum transferrin   mg/%
      Cholesterol   Mmo1/1
   3. Inmunologic response parameters
      Total lymphocyte count
      Skin test antigens (Streptokinase+Urokinase, Candida,
      Tricophiton, Toxoplasmine, Tuberculine.

(Streptokinase + Urokinase, Candida, Tricophyton,
Toxoplasmine, Tuberculin) are included.
        The P.N.I. was calculated according to Mullen et
al.(1980). This formula relates four nutritional status
parameters (S.Albumin, S.Transferrin, Triceps skinfold and
Immunologic response) (Table 7).
        Parenteral or enteral nutrition was ordered
depending of nutritional status, daily caloric requirements,
degree of dysphagia and tolerance to oral feeding before
surgery.
        Three patients received parenteral nutrition
before surgery. Two of them by peripheral route as a
complement of their oral nutrition during 6 days. The third
patient received T.P.N. during 13 days due to a total
dysphagia. Data related with parenteral
nutrition in these patients are shown in Table 8.
        Postoperative T.P.N. was administered to all

TABLE 7: CALCULATION OF PROGNOSTIC NUTRITIONAL INDEX(P.N.I)

%P.N.I.= 158%-(16.8 x S.Albumin(gr/dl))-(0.76 x Triceps
         skinfold (mm))-(0.2 x S.Transferrin (mg/dl))-
         -(5.8 skin tests)*
 *= Skin test: Not response= 0
         Induration<5mm to one or more antigens= 1
         Induration>5mm to one or more antigens= 2

patients. Data on this are shown in Table 8.

Beforehand, net protein utilization (Blackburn,G.
1977) and basal energy expenditure according to Benedit were
calculated to ensure correct nitrogen and calories
administration.

Usual controls for patients receiving T.P.N.
established in our protocols were followed with these
patients.

Finally, we collected data retrospectively on all
postoperative complications in these patients.

Complications were divided in surgical and non
surgical and these in septic and non septic.(Tables 9.1/9.2)

RESULTS

Studying preoperative nutritional status of the
patients we observed (Fig.1) a severe protein-calorie
malnutrition (60%) in fat pool (7 patients had a little
triceps skinfold) and moderate (60-90%) in protein pool(arm
muscle circumference and creatinine/height index).

At the same time some protein malnutrition
parameters were also modified as can be seen in Fig.2.

The preoperative P.N.I. found is shown in Table 10.

Three patients had a P.N.I. lower than 50%, 3
patients between 50-60% and 4 patients higher than 60%.

Postoperative complications occurred in a high
percentage. (Table 11.1 and 11.2).Only one patient had no
complications.

The most frequent complication was wound dehiscence
that was severe in 5 patients leading to **mediastinitis**

TABLE 8: PREOPERATIVE PARENTERAL NUTRITION

N.P.	N.Pat.	N.Days	Kcal/Kg/Day	GN_2/Kg/Day	Non Prot.Cal:GN_2
Peripheral	2	6	33	0.138	1:146
Central	1	13	46	0.262	1:175

POSTOPERATIVE PARENTERAL NUTRITION

Central	10	18 ± 11	36 ± 5.4	0.22 ± 0.033	$1:159\pm6$

TABLE 9.1 POSTOPERATIVE COMPLICATIONS

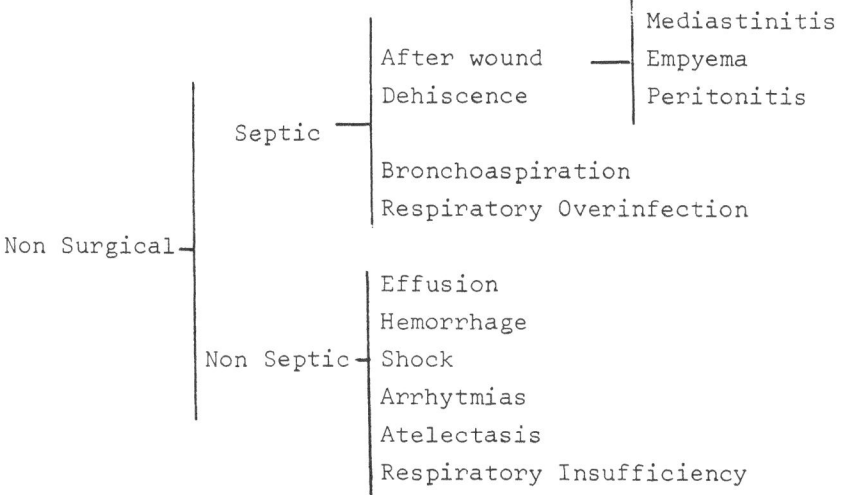

Surgical
- Wound Dehiscence — Severe / Mild
- Acute Hemorrhage
- Perforation
- Eventration

TABLE 9.2: POSTOPERATIVE COMPLICATIONS

Non Surgical
- Septic
  - After wound Dehiscence — Mediastinitis / Empyema / Peritonitis
  - Bronchoaspiration
  - Respiratory Overinfection
- Non Septic
  - Effusion
  - Hemorrhage
  - Shock
  - Arrhytmias
  - Atelectasis
  - Respiratory Insufficiency

TABLE 10: PATIENT DISTRIBUTION ACCORDING TO PREOPERATIVE PNI

P.N.I.	N.PATIENTS
<50%	3
50-60%	3
>60%	4

TABLE 11.1RELATION BETWEEN POSTOP.COMPLICATIONS AND P.N.I.

Complications Surgical		P.N.I. $<$50%	P.N.I. $>$50%	TOTAL
Wound dehiscence	Severe	0	5	5
	Mild	3	0	3
Acute Hemorrhage		0	1	1
Perforation		0	1	1
Eventration		0	1	1
No Surgical				
Septic				
Empyema		0	2	2
Mediastinitis		0	2	2
Peritonitis		0	2	2
Bronchoaspiration		0	2	2
Pneumonia		0	2	2

TABLE 11.2 RELATION BETWEEN POSTOP.COMPLICATIONS AND P.N.I.

Complications No Surgical	$<$50%	P.N.I. $>$50%	TOTAL
No Septic			
Respiratory Insufficiency	2	2	4
Quilotorax	1	0	1
Effusion	2	1	3
Atelectasis	0	1	1
Arrhythmias	0	2	2

N.Of complications with P.N.I. $<$50% = 8
N.Of complications with P.N.I. $>$50% =24
Reoperations = 3 Patients with P.N.I. $>$ 50%
Hospital Postoperative mortality: 2 patients with P.N.I.$>$50%
Total complications: 32

abdominal or pleural sepsis and less severe in 3 patients.
        In another case a iatrogenic gastric perforation
occurred.
        Observing non surgical septic complications the
most relevant were 2 bronchoaspiration and 2 pneumonia.

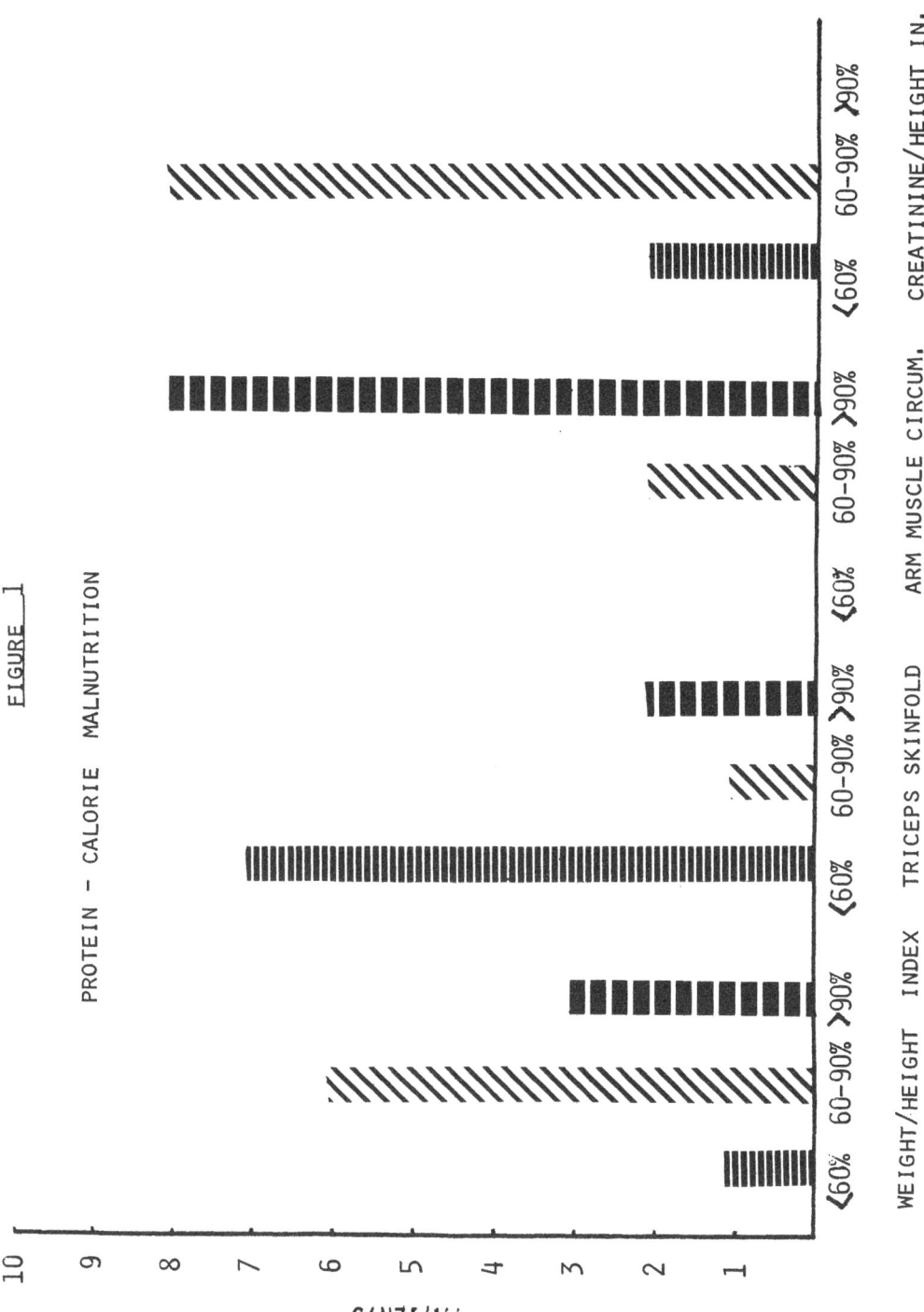

FIGURE 1

PROTEIN – CALORIE MALNUTRITION

FIGURE 2

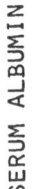

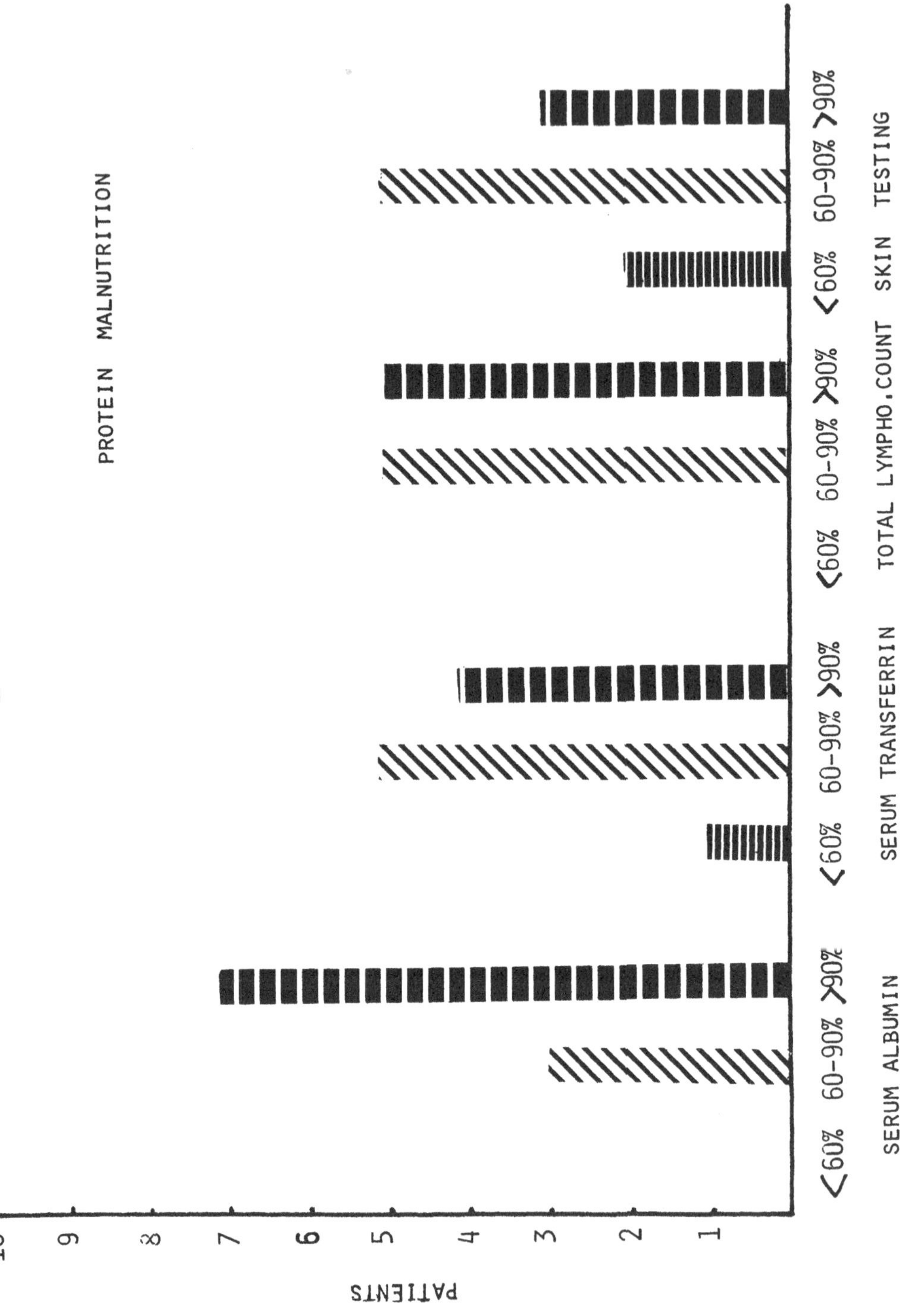
PROTEIN MALNUTRITION
PATIENTS
10
9
8
7
6
5
4
3
2
1
<60% 60-90% >90%
SERUM ALBUMIN
<60% 60-90% >90%
SERUM TRANSFERRIN
<60% 60-90% >90%
TOTAL LYMPHO.COUNT
<60% 60-90% >90%
SKIN TESTING

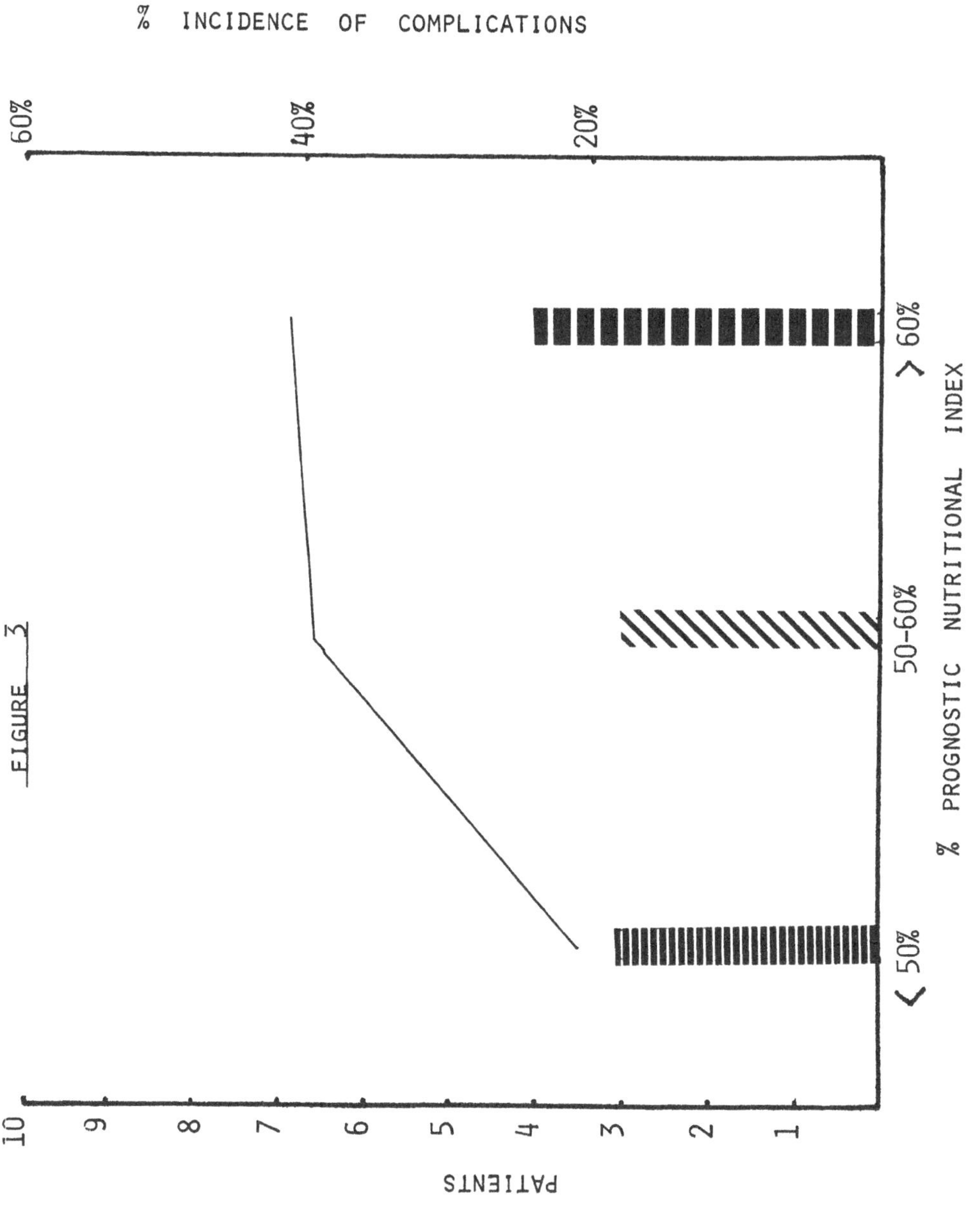
% INCIDENCE OF COMPLICATIONS
60%
40%
20%
PATIENTS
10
9
8
7
6
5
4
3
2
1
< 50%
50-60%
> 60%
% PROGNOSTIC NUTRITIONAL INDEX

FIGURE 3

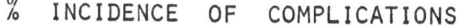

TABLE 12:

P.N.I	N.PAT.	COMPLICATIONS WITHOUT	COMPLICATIONS WITH	COMPLICATIONS SURG.	COMPLICATIONS NO SURG.	HOSP.POST. MORTALITY	REOPERATIVE
⟨50%	3	-	3	3	3	-	-
⟩50%	7	1	6	6	5	2	3
TOTAL	10	1	9	9	8	2	3

Non septic complications observed were 3 effusion, 1 atelectasis, 2 arrhythmias following a mediastinitis and 4 respiratory insufficiency.

Three patients had to be reoperated and the hospital postoperative mortality was 20%.

Looking for a relation between P.N.I. and postoperative complications we found that 20,5% of complications occurred in patients with a P.N.I. lower than 50%, 38,5% in patients with a P.N.I. between 50 and 60% and 41% in patients with a P.N.I. higher than 60%. (Fig. 3).

Observing that patients with a P.N.I. higher than 50% had an 80% of incidence complications we divided patients in two groups: patients with a P.N.I. higher 50% and patients with a P.N.I. lower than 50%.

In the group of patients with P.N.I. lower than 50%, in spite of complications occurred they were mild. No patients had to be reoperated and no patients died.

Among the 7 patients with a P.N.I. higher than 50% one patient had no complications but 6 patients had severe surgical complications and 5 of them had also non surgical complications. Three patients had to be reoperated and two patients died. (Table 12)

No technic or metabolic complications occurred neither in preoperative nor in the postoperative due to parenteral nutrition.

CONCLUSIONS

-We think that P.N.I. can be a useful parameter to evaluate patients with carcinoma of esophagus in the preoperative.

-In spite of the small number of patients studied, we have found   a relation between P.N.I. and the number of postoperative complications.

When the P.N.I. is higher than 50%, the number of postoperative complications occurred in our patients was higher and they are more severe.

-All patients with carcinoma of esophagus who arrive to the hospital to undergo surgery are candidates for preoperative parenteral nutrition.

-Due to the small number of patients included, we decided to continue the study in order to get a larger sample to be able to obtain more significative conclusions.

REFERENCES

Akiyama,H.(1980).Surgery for carcinoma of the esophagus.Curr. Probl.Surg.February.

Alastrué,A.et al.(1982).Parámetros antropométricos en nuestra población.Bol.SENPE,no.4:3-18.

Appelquist,P.(1972).Carcinoma of the esophagus and gastric cardies. A retrospective study based on statistical and clinical material from Finland.Acta Chirurgica Scandinava (Suppl.).430:1-86.

Blackburn,G. et al.(1977).Nutritional and metabolic asessment of the hospitalized patient. JPEN,no.1:11-22.

Mc.Keown,K.C.(1981).Resection of Midesophageal Carcinoma with esophagogastric anastomosis.World.J.Surg.no5:517-525

Moertel,C.G.(1973).The Esophagus.Cancer Medecine.J.F.Holland and E.Frei III.Eds.Philadelphia.Lea & Febiger,pp. 1519-1526.

Mullen,J.L. et al.(1980).Reduction of operative morbidity and mortality by combined preoperative and postoperative nutritional support.Ann.Surg.192 no.5:604-613.

Nakayama,K.et al(1967).Surgical treatment combined with preoperative irradiation for esophageal cancer. Cancer 20:778-788.

Ong,G.B.(1971).Resection and reconstruction of the esophagus

Curr.Probl.Surg.September.

Prieto Lorenzo,A.(1976).Mortalidad por tumores malignos en
        España (1951-1970).Ministerio de Gobernación.
        Dirección General de Sanidad.Madrid.

CENTRAL NERVOUS SYSTEM (CNS) PROPHYLAXIS OF ACUTE LYMPHOBLASTIC
LEUKEMIA (ALL) WITH METHOTREXATE (MTX).

M.J.M. Oosterbaan[1],R.J.J.Lippens[2],B.Winograd[1],T.B.Vree[1] and
E. van der Kleijn[1].

1 Department of Clinical Pharmacy
2 Department of pediatrics, Sint Radboud Hospital,
   University of Nijmegen, Nijmegen, The Netherlands.

Introduction.

The treatment of the subclinical manifestations of acute lymphoblastic
leukemia (ALL) of the central nervous system is called CNS-prophylaxis,
which consists of radiotherapy (cranial irradiation) and administrations
of methotrexate (MTX). The objectives of the treatment are a delay of the
clinical symtoms associated with CNS-leukemia for about 1 to 5 years or
even longer.

To obtain a concentration of 5×10^{-7} Mol/L in the cerebrospinal fluid for
a period of time, long enough to be effective (18 hours), the antimetabolite MTX is administered as high dose infusions or intralumbarly.

A third way to achieve high enough concentrations makes use of a drain
in the ventricular space, called Ommaya reservoir.

After some remarks on the pharmacokinetics in general, the above mentioned
three methods of administration will be discussed in more detail.

Pharmacokinetics of methotrexate.

In Figure 1 the plasma concentrations versus time are shown from a patient
treated with MTX by means of an i.v. bolus injection. The plasma concentration-time profile can be described by a two exponential function. This
can be visualized by a two compartment model. The first compartment represents the plasma compartment, from which the concentrations are determined.
The second compartment represents that volume of the body in which MTX is
distributed, but cannot be measured. This means no physiological equivalent can be found for this abstract compartment. The half life of the
first exponential is 70 min., that of the second 5 h and 26 min. The distribution volume of the central compartment V_1 accounts for 30 L, which
suggests a distribution over blood and into the extracellular volume.

MTX is metabolized to 7-OH-MTX, from which the plasma concentration-time
curve is shown. This runs parallel to that of MTX. The main route of

elimination for MTX as well as for 7-OH-MTX is renal excretion. About 90% of the administered dose can be recovered from urine. The renal clearance of MTX of this patient was measured to be 150 ml/min.

When MTX is administered by means of an infusion a more or less stable steady state concentration can be achieved during the period of the infusion. Peak plasma concentrations that do not contribute to, or are even dangerous for the treatment are avioded.

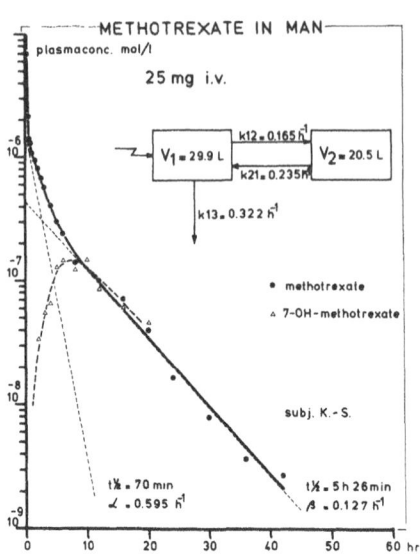

High dose infusions.

With a high dose infusion, i.e. 3 g MTX/m^2, plasma concentrations of 1 x 10^{-3} Mol/L are achieved. Animal studies elucidated that the ratio of plasma concentration: CSF concen-

Figure 1. Plasma concentration profile in a patient after an i.v. bolus injection. The plasma concentration of the metabolite 7-OH-MTX is also shown.

tration is in the range of 30:1. In patients this ratio was observed to be in the same range, from 30 to 80., as calculated from plasma and CSF samples which were drawn at the same time. This means, that if one wants to obtain a minimum concentration of 5 x 10^{-7} Mol/L in the CSF for a period of 18 hours, a 30 to 80 times higher concentration of 1.5 to 4.0 x 10^{-5} Mol/L in plasma has to be maintained during a period of 24 hours; based on 18 hours treatment and 6 hours to reach the state of equilibrium between the plasma compartment and the CSF compartment. With the aid of the pharmacokinetic parameters, the required dosage to maintain this plasma concentration can be calculated. Assuming linear kinetics, the calculated dosage amounts to 1.5 10 4.0 mg/h.kg. For a child of 20 kg this means a total dosage of 0.7 to 1.9 g MTX.

Intralumbal injections.

In the applied treatment protocols the lumbal injections of MTX are used as the only way of administration in the CSF-prophylaxis. In a period of 2.5 weeks 5 intralumbal injections are given. Yen et al (1978) measured the loss of ^{3}H-MTX from the spinal cord into the blood compartment after intraventricular, percutaneous lumbar or spinal catheter administration.

The lumbal injection causes a high loss of ^{3}H-MTX into the blood, whereas
the loss after the other two administrations is low. These findings
strongly suggest a loss through the lumbar sac which has a good blood
supply. From a pharmacokinetic point of view, this mode of administration
can be compared with an oral administration, the lumbar region represen-
ting now the intestine from which MTX is absorbed into the blood compartment. Lippens (1981) shows the plasma concentration-time profiles of five
subsequent intralumbal injections (Figure 2). The plasma concentration-
time profiles resemble the ones after oral administration. It can be seen
that the profile changes with increasing number of injections. This phenomenon can be simulated by altering the absorption rate constant of a
two compartment model keeping the rate constant of distribution and elimination constant. The physiological meaning of the increased exsorption
from CSF into blood may be   mechanical damage, due to the injection or
   chemical damage due to MTX,   both may allow a faster release from
the lumbar region into the blood. The plasma concentration-time profiles
after intralumbal injections change from a 'slow absorption type' into
a 'fast absorption type'.

From Figure 2 it is anticipa-
ted that only the first two
injections can deliver MTX
to the regions where it is
required. The 3rd, 4th and
5th injection probably will
not contribute to achieve
MTX concentrations in the
cerebrospinal fluid sur-
rounding the brain. To
study the distribution from
the lumbar sac to the ventricular space by distribution properties of the CSF
and diffusion mechanisms
in the spinal cord, Tc^{99m}
was administered together
with the MTX intralumbarly.
The radioactivity was measured at 4 locations alongside

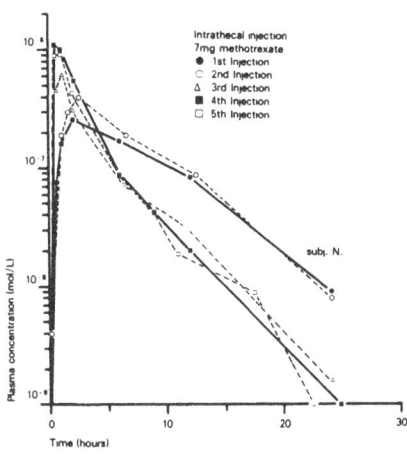

*Figure 2. Methotrexate plasma concentrations
in a child after each of 5 subsequent intralumbal injections, showing the 2 different
types of plasma disappearance curves.*

the spinal cord at different time intervals. A gradually decreasing radio-activity going up the spinal cord can be observed. Only 5% of the radio-activity measured at the place of administration reaches the large cis-terns. The main difference of the distribution between the first and the fourth injection is the higher concentration of radioactivity in the lower part of the spinal cord. This is in agreement with the observation of the fast type exsorption in plasma, which was verified by measuring radioactivity in plasma, being 4 times higher 30 minutes after the fourth administration as compared to the first. At the moment we are studying whether an increased interval between two intralumbal injections, i.e. from ½ week to 1 or 2 weeks, results in plasma concentration-time profiles of the slow type only. Preliminary observations show no differences be-tween ½ week and 1 week intervals. Only the first two injections were observed to be of the slow type. However, all 2 week interval injections show a release of MTX into the blood. So within 2 weeks the repair of the mechanical and/or chemical damage has been completed.

Intraventricular injections.
Application of MTX via an Ommaya reservoir is obviously the best way to obtain high enough MTX concentrations in the CSF around the hemispheres. Concentrations of more than 1×10^{-5} Mol/L are obtained using a dosage of 0.5 mg MTX. U. Bode (1981) demonstrates that MTX is rapidly cleared from the CSF, but for a period of 15 hours the concentration stays above the required concentration of 5×10^{-7} Mol/L. Bleyer et al (1978) introduced a Concentration x Time (CxT) therapy, which means a therapy in which the CSF concentration of MTX can be maintained above 5×10^{-7} Mol/L for about 72 hours. The intraventricular administrations of 1 mg MTX with inter-vals of 12 hours result in a more or less stable CSF concentration. In his study he compared the efficacy and toxicity of patients treated with the CxT therapy and with a single intraventricular injection. No differen-ces were observed in rate of remission induction, the number of relapses or the duration of the remission. However, he also concluded that because of the lower cumulative dosage used in the CxT group, 66 versus 173 mg MTX, the CxT therapy is less neurotoxic.

Conclusion.
From a pharmacokinetic point of view, the best way to perform CNS-prophy-laxis is the administration of MTX by means of an Ommaya reservoir. As the

ethical problems associated with this kind of administration are of the same magnitude compared to the other ways of administration, the CxT therapy of Bleyer, resulting in a lower neurotoxicity is preferable. When intralumbal injections are used, they have to be spaced at two weeks inter·vals to obtain the maximum effect.

References.

Bleyer,W.A.,Poplack,D.G. and Simon,R.M. (1978). "Concentration x Time" methotrexate via a subcutaneous reservoir: A less toxic regimen for intraventricular chemotherapy of central nervous system neoplasms. Blood 51 ,5,835-842.

Bode,U. (1981) Methotrexatpharmakokinetik in menschlichem liquor. Universitätsklinik Bonn.

Lippens,R.J.J. (1981) Methotrexate in the central nervous system prophylaxis of children with acute lymphoblastic leukemia. Thesis, University of Nijmegen, The Netherlands.

Yen,J, Reis,F.L., Kimelberg,H.K.and Bourke,R.S. (1978) Direct administration of methotrexate into the central nervous system of primates. J. Neurosurg. 48, 895-902.

THE TREATMENT PROTOCOLS OF ACUTE LYMPHOBLASTIC LEUKEMIA
IN CHILDREN

R.J.J. Lippens and G.A.M. de Vaan
Department of Pediatrics,
Sint Radboud Hospital, University of Nijmegen,
Geert Grooteplein Zuid 20,
6525 GA Nijmegen,
The Netherlands.

The era of chemotherapy for acute lymphoblastic leukemia (ALL)[3]
began in 1948 when Farber introduced aminopterin and obtained temporary
remissions. Before that time, children with acute leukemia had a median
survival of about 2-4 months. The only support that could be given was
blood transfusion. During the next 10 years three other agents were introduced: methotrexate, 6-mercaptopurine and corticosteroids, resulting in a
remission rate of respectively 26, 22 and 63% for single drugs, resulting
in a median survival of 6-12 months[1]. In the next decade cyclophosphamide,
vincristin, cytosine arabinoside, daunorubicin and l-asparaginase were
found to induce remissions as single agents. In the treatment of ALL some
agents are more effective than others, but currently no drug is used as a
single agent for the purpose of inducing a remission.
An intensive search for finding the most optimal treatment method of ALL
was done in the St. Jude Childrens Research Hospital in Memphis, resulting
in 1966 in the so-called "Total Therapy"[5].
The purpose of the treatment schedule was meant to have the intention of
curative therapy. Total therapy has always included:
1. remission induction therapy
2. "prophylactic" treatment of the central nervous system (CNS)
3. continuation of the treatment by a maintenance therapy
When this concept was developed it was not yet clear, and in fact it is
still not clear, if the main point of treatment should be accentuated on
the induction or the maintenance treatment.
The purpose of this remission induction treatment is to reach as fast and
as efficiently as possible a complete remission of the bone marrow, with
as little as possible side-effects.

The occurrence of CNS-leukemia is prevented (i.e. destroying subclinical leukemic invasions in the meninges) with a treatment early in the hematologic remission (CNS-prophylaxis). This treatment consists of irradiation of the CNS (cranial only or craniospinal irradiation) and/ or intrathecal administration of cytostatics.

The moment of CNS-prophylaxis will be discussed. The largest cell-kill in the CNS-area should also be obtained as soon as possible in the beginning of the induction treatment. The agents used in this induction treatment will not pass the blood-brain barrier sufficiently, so no contribution to the treatment of subclinical invasion of the meninges can be expected from the cytostatics administered intravenously in the remission induction treatment.

At last subclinical residual leukemic cell populations are destroyed by a combination of drugs during 2-3 years.

ALL is subdivided into two groups, depending on the signs and symptoms of the disease at presentation. The "standard-risk" ALL initiates with a relatively small number of leukocytes in the blood, the "high-risk" ALL has a large number of leukocytes in the blood (etc.). Discussion exists on the number of leukocytes defining standard-or high-risk leukemia.

A typical induction treatment scheme of standard-risk ALL may consist of weekly i.v. injections of vincristin and daily administration of prednisone Together with the 5th injection of vincristin a 14-days course of asparaginase is given (fig.1).

			INDUCTION	MAINTENANCE
Cranial irradiation				
MTX-Pred. 12.5 mg/m²		i.th.		
VCR	2 mg/m²/w	i.v.		
Pred.	40 mg/m²/d	or.		
L-ASP	200 E/kg/d	im/i.v.		
6-MP	50 mg/m²/d	or.		
MTX	30 mg/m²/w	or.		
BM				
LP+i.t. MTX-Pred.				
		weeks	0 2 4 6 8	10 12 14 16 18 20 22 24 26 28 30 32

Fig.1: Treatment protocol in standard-risk A.L.L.
(Abbreviations see Fig. 2)

All patients receive a CNS-prophylactic treatment. In high-risk ALL the basic pattern of treatment is the same as in standard-risk ALL. However, cyclophosphamide and adriamycin are added to the protocol (fig.2).

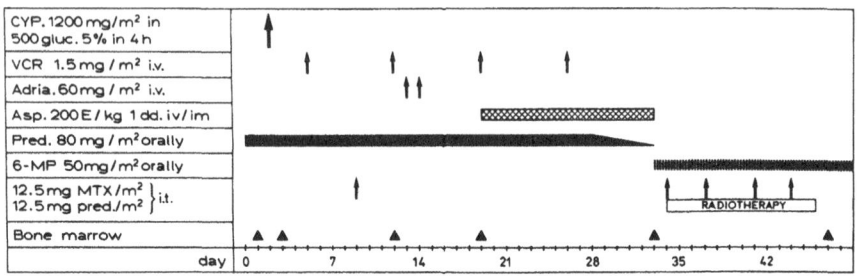

Fig.2: Treatment protocol in high-risk A.L.L.

CYP=Cyclophosphamide   VCR=Vincristin   Adria=Adriamycin
ASP=l-Asparaginase   Pred=Prednisone   6-MP =6-Mercaptopurine
MTX=Methotrexate

The treatment regimen in ALL is composed of traditional combinations of drugs. Other methods of treatment might be as effective, but it is not very attractive to change protocols which have rather good results.

We have studied the action of adriamycin in children with high-risk ALL[4]. According to the protocol, adriamycin was given at two subsequent days with a daily dose of 60 mg/m^2. Although the antileukemic action appeared to be satisfactory, the toxicity on bone marrow and gastrointestinal tract was considerable and 6 of 16 children have died of severe gastrointestinal toxicity, culminating in an irreversible shock (not caused by the cardiotoxic action of adriamycin). Pharmacokinetic studies (M. Oosterbaan) showed that the peak concentration of the second dose of adriamycin was 60-times higher than in the first dose. These peak concentrations are considered to be the cause of the serious toxicity. By giving the complete dose of two days together in one infusion (120 mg/m^2) during 24 hours,

the distribution and elimination of adriamycin showed a constant concentration level, as high as the concentration level of the bolus injection
in the β-phase. This concentration level is responsible for the desired
antitumor action. By using these 24-hours infusions of adriamycin in 14
children, there were no further deaths attributable to adriamycin. Side-
effects to bone marrow and digestive tract have become mild The action
on cell-kill, however, is unknown yet. Until now we have not observed a
change in the remission-rate and the duration of the remission in these
children, comparing 24-hours infusions with the 2 subsequent bolus injections of adriamycin.

Following every hematologic remission, children with ALL undergo a CNS-prophylactic treatment consisting of cranial irradiation (2500 R)
during 2,5 weeks. In this period 5 intralumbar injections with methotraxate
and prednisolone (both 12.5 mg/m^2) are given. This treatment causes a number of side-effects[2]: ulcerative lesions of the digestive tract, especially
the mucosa of the mouth, resulting in a sometimes severe anorexia and
weight loss; and depression of the bone marrow resulting in leukopenia (16%
of the children), thrombocytopenia (16%) and anemia (30%), requiring blood
transfusions. These side-effects, although not life-threatening, hamper the
children in their convalescence. The side-effects are attributed to the
action of methotrexate. However, the dose used in the CNS-prophylaxis with
a maximum of 15 mg, is rather small. In the maintenance treatment of ALL a
dose of 30 mg/m^2 is used during 2 years once a week without side-effects.
This makes the phenomenon observed during the CNS-prophylaxis difficult to
understand. Moreover, we observed a failure of the CNS-prophylaxis in 26%
of the children, resulting in an overt CNS-leukemia 73 weeks (median interval) after diagnosis. In high-risk ALL patients the incidence of CNS-leukemia appears to be even 45%. Although the expression of the ALL in these
children may have a more aggressive character, the unsatisfactory results
might also be influenced by an insufficient action of methotrexate. This
problem could be understood by pharmacokinetic studies of methotrexate following intrathecal injections[2].

1. George M, Hernandez K, Husto O, Borrella L, Holton C, Pinkel D. A study of "total therapy" of acute lymphocytic leukemia in children. J. Pediatrics 1968, 72: 399-408.
2. Lippens RJJ. Methotrexate in the central nervous system prophylaxis of children with acute lymphoblastic leukemia. Thesis Nijmegen 1981.
3. Mauer AM. Therapy of acute lymphoblastic leukemia in childhood. Blood 1980, 56: 1-10.
4. Oosterbaan MJM, Dirks MJM, Vree TB, Van der Kleijn E, Simonetti GS, McVie JG. Klinische farmacokinetiek van Adriamycine. Tijds. Geneesm. Onderzoek. 1982, 7: 1372-1378.
5. Pinkel D. Five year follow-up of "total therapy" of childhood lymphocytic leukemia. J. Amer. Med. Ass. 1971, 216: 648-652.

GUIDELINES FOR THE SAFE HANDLING OF CYTOTOXIC DRUGS -
WITH SPECIAL EMPHASIS ON THE USE OF MINIBAGS

K.Wågen, Pharm. M. Sci.
Pharmaceutical Department
N-9012 Regionsykehuset i Tromsø, Norway

Norway is still like an underdeveloped country in the field
of hospital or clinical pharmacy. It is therefore like
crossing a new border when you succeed in your efforts to
improve.   What I am now going to tell you may therefore
sound like a blast from the past, but I do want to show you
that not all your members work under excellent conditions,
but that you may improve in spite of them.

Our pharmaceutical department has two pharmacists
covering distribution, information and control on the wards,
a third covering control in nursing homes - more than 30
spread over an area of appr. 20.000 sqkm. The department
was to undergo an enlargement just as Norway had regulations
for the handling of cytotoxic drugs. We used the opportunity
to build facilities for centralized admixture service, to
which the administrators of the hospital were very positive.
The content of the regulations have been given to you in
Stresa last year and will not be repeated here.

With the facilities and personnel, we had few
problems in selling our service to the wards. I here must
add that the hospital has no oncology unit, the patients are
spread on several wards depending on the location of the
cancer. In addition those needing radiotherapy are sent to
Oslo. A majority of the patients are found on one medical
ward. We also have large polyclinics and treat some cancer
patients there.

The use of minibags for antibiotics is well known in
the hospital. When we offered the service of reconstituting
cytotoxics, we simultaneously tried a shift from the use of
syringes to using minibags.

Our arguments for it were:
- safer handling
- less risk of extravasation
- reduction in nausea and vomiting

The physicians were at first sceptical,the main argument
being the time aspect. In Norway the practice is for the
physician to give cytotoxics. The fear of minibags increasing administration time and thus taking more of his/her
time were therefore important to them.

At this time the hospital was in the lucky position
of having employed a nurse whose task is to care for the
cancer patients and try to solve their physical and social
problems. She supported us and we got the physicians to try.
Let me add that a lot of the physicians had nothing against
using minibags. After a short time trial in the internal
polyclinic, the physicians and the patients were enthusias-
tic, and we were asked to use minibags for all the patients.

To order cytotoxic drugs, the physician has to fill
in a special order sheet or telephone. Due to transportation problems because the pharmacy is located outside the
main building, several orders are made by phonecalls. We
hoped, when we started, to get the orders at least one day
ahead, but can never rely on that. Therefore we most frequently have to prepare immediately after order is received.
On average we reconstitute 6 - 7 drugs/day for approximately
3 patients.

After checking by the pharmacist, technicians fill
in labels, the patient card and do the reconstituting.

For each drug we keep a card giving the necessary
information on reconstitution, storage, stability and special
precautions. In addition we keep a record of the patients.
The wards have access to the same information through sheets
on each drug which, in addition to the information on our
cards, give indications, usual dosage, side effects and
contraindications. There are also procedures on administration, handling of waste, treatment of extravasation etc.

The preparation is done in a laminar   flow hood.

As often as possible reconstitution is done directly into plastic bags. Today only two drugs need glass container.

The drugs for one patient are labelled, packed and delivered to the ward. Altogether one delivery consists of the drugs, a signed copy of the order sheet and an administration set.

The drugs are administered via a Y-set where one branch is connected with a sodium chloride bag of 250 - 1000 ml. This bag is used to control position of the venflon cannulae, to flush ad libitum during the administration of the drugs and afterwards. The bag may contain an antiemetic. Waste is handled in accordance with written instructions.

What is our experience:
- Travenol offers extensive information on the storage of cytotoxics in Viaflex plastic containers - information which are lacking when you use syringes.
- Reconstitution is done in a closed system and under laminair flow giving protection of personnel and minimal danger of microbial contamination.
- Infusion via a Y-set is a safe and easy procedure.
- The patients experience less nausea and vomiting, those having tried both ask for the bags.

There are many trials going on around the world regarding cancer treatment, the combination of drugs, the size of the dose, length of the course, the number of courses, infusion time etc. What we offer now is an alternative to syringes - discussions on for example increasing infusion time to reduce nausea is a decision for the physician.

Clinical pharmacy is a neglected field in Norway due to lack of pharmacists, but also to the lack of postgraduate education possibilities and interest in involvement which may lead to long or shifting working hours. By centralizing the preparation of cytotoxic drugs we have brought back to the pharmacy a galenical preparation which has been carried out by non-pharmaceutical personnel.

In addition it has given us closer contact with physicians, nurses and patients. We have acquired extensive knowledge in the field and are now able to discuss on more equal terms and focus on specific problems.

In our hospital it was natural to let the pharmacy do the reconstitution. In other hospitals which have an oncology unit it will be natural to place it there.

CENTRALIZATION OF PREPARATION OF CYTOTOXIC DRUGS IN THE
CENTRAL PHARMACY : ONE YEAR OF EXPERIENCE

Léon WILMOTTE, Cliniques Universitaires Saint-Luc,
1200 Bruxelles, Belgium

The high local toxicity of cytotoxic drugs (skin, mucous membranes, ...) is well known. Important precautionary measures must be taken while handling these drugs in order to avoid any contact with the skin. Difficulties associated with obligatory precision of dosages implies a risk of error, very detrimental to the patient.
Recent studies suggest that a potential additional hazard of carcinogenicity exists for the personnel handling repeatedly these drugs without sufficient care.

For all these reasons, it seemed interesting to examine the possibility to centralize their handling in the central Pharmacy.
Our goal was double :
- to demonstrate the quality improvement of patient treatment and the security of the preparator.
- to prove time and procedures savings with this centralization.

Because the experiment had to be done without any additional personnel and still had to be significant, we selected Pneumology and Urology Units, for several reasons :
- These Units use 22,3 % of total consumption of cytotoxic drugs in our hospital.
- The Medical and Nursing staffs were interested in the study.
- The treatments are essentially administred during the day and can be easy scheduled in the daily workload of the Pharmacy.

First quarter 82

Oncology	2.838 vials	50,7 %
Pneumology	890 vials	16 %
General Medicine	617 vials	11,2 %
Urology	354 vials	6,3 %
Aseptic Unit	347 vials	6,2 %
Hematology	268 vials	4,7 %
Pediatric Unit	160 vials	2,8 %
Varia	118 vials	2,1 %

In order to assure sufficient safety for our personnel, we adopted the following guidelines :
- use of a vertical laminar flow containment hood
- wearing gloves and protective garments
- use of equipment to avoid or reduce splashing at the time of reconstitution
- work done by an experienced hospital pharmacist until a technician is trained for this task.

A particular prescription form was designed, with mention of :

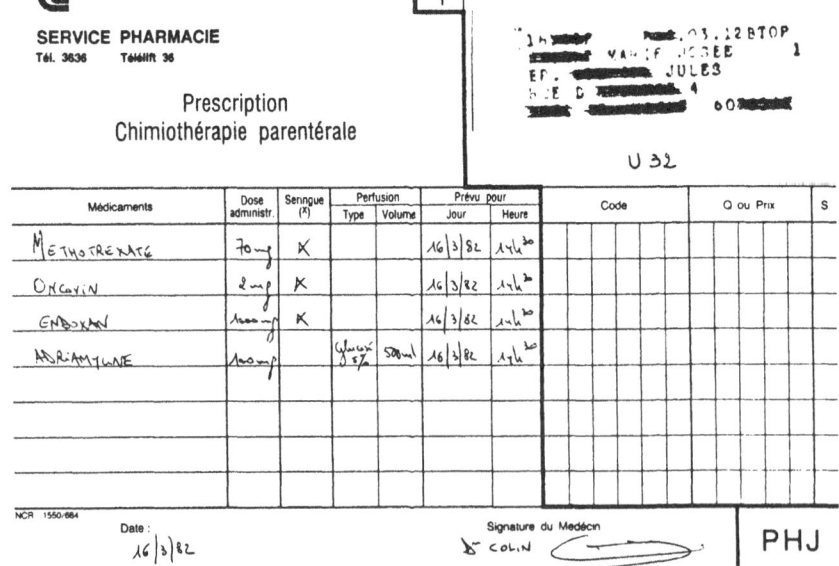

- the name of the drug
- the dose to be administred
- the way of administration : syringe or infusion (type, volume)
- the time of administration to the patient
- the identification of the patient

A label recapitulating these data and the moment of preparation has to be stuck   on the syringe or the infusion.

The experiment started on July 1981.
After one year, a comparative evaluation of the procedures used in the Pharmacy and in the Pneumology Unit was realised. A pharmacist, not directly involved in the study, made a detailed observation of the course of preparations during two weeks in the ward and two weeks in the Pharmacy.

After submission to the physicians and medical nurses, the conclusions were approved by them.

QUANTITATIVE FINDINGS
_____

A comparison was made of the time spent for the reconstitutions in the Pharmacy and on the ward. In the latter case, two times are
sometimes noted : real time including disturbances and reconstitution
time properly. In the case of reconstitutions of one to two vials, there
is no significant difference of time.

| Prescription | Number of vials | Number of minutes on ward | | Number of minutes in the Pharmacy |
		including disturbance	handling only	
Platinol 130 to 160 mg in NaCl 0,9 % 150 ml	13 to 16	25 to 35	25 to 27	15 to 20
Vincristine 1 mg and 2 mg (syringe)	1 to 2		4 to 5	3 to 4
Cyclophosphamide 500 mg	1		6	5
1 g	2	20	10	5
Adriamycin 100 mg	10		30	16 to 17
Vindesine 5 mg	1		2	3 to 5
First quarter 82	890		46 hours	28 hours

On the other hand, when a dozen or more of vials are implicated
(eg. Platinol vial 10 mg, Adriblastina vial 10 mg), an important difference
appears systematically (25 minutes in the ward, 15 minutes in the Pharmacy). Furthermore, reconstitution in series of drugs with sufficient stability would allow additional time saving (eg. Bleomycin).

QUALITATIVE FINDINGS
_____

a) Equipment used

There are few differences between equipment commonly used in
the ward and in the Pharmacy.
Two facts must still be noted :
   - use by the Pharmacy of vented needles that allow removal of   pres-
     sure and so avoid splashing during reconstitution.

- interaction between the hospital pharmacist and the pharmaceutical
  industry resulting in modifications of dosage forms. For example,
  the design of some vials did not allow a total emptying of their
  content. Modifications of plugs resolved the problem. Users in the
  ward had never before mentioned these defects.

b) Work environment

In the ward, cytotoxic drugs were prepared in the drug room as
all the other drugs. This room has no special ventilation. Splatterings
   fall on the tables and the floor. Other drugs, injectable or oral, are
simultaneously prepared on the same table top.
The nurse is often disturbed by the telephone, various requests, tasks to
accomplish at definite times (take blood samples, blood pressure, ...).
This is prejudicial to the quality of the preparation.
The environment in the Pharmacy, as described above, warrants better
conditions regarding intellectual concentration and hygiene.

c) Protection of the preparator

Nursing and medical students do not appear to be sufficiently
sensitive to the risk of topical contact by these drugs.
For economical reasons, gloves used by nurses are "one size" P.V.C.
gloves. Handling is not easy. The nurses prefers to work more carefully,
barehanded. Three times, during the two weeks of observation time, nurses
spilled drugs on their hands (Vincristine, Adriamycin   Platinol). They
did not wash their hands before completion of their task. Some had meanwhile taken the telephone or touched other things. The reconstitution
equipment used does not follow any special process of elimination.
In the Pharmacy, the preparator wears an overgarment with long sleeves
as well as adjusted size gloves that he can keep for the whole series of
operations. His eyes and lungs are protected by a glass wall and the vertical laminar flow. Perceptible projections on this glass prove that the
wearing of glasses in the ward is not superfluous. The table top and the
walls of the laminar flow hood are cleaned with an antiseptic solution
before and after each sequence of preparations.
Equipment used (syringes, compresses, ...) is eliminated in special
yellow closed bags in order to avoid any subsequent contact during the
waste evacuation.

d) Asepsis of the preparation

        Some errors of asepsis were currently noted in the ward :
- a bad disinfection of the plugs before puncture
- non sterile air systematically injected into the vials.

These wrong handlings have been avoided in the Pharmacy by :
- the use of a laminar flow hood
- the awareness of the preparator to the quality of his manipulations.

e) Accuracy of the dosage

        Several cases of overdosage have been noted, although the
nurse knew she was observed :
- spilling of drug out of the vial, causing a loss of 25 %
- serial reconstitutions with a single volume of diluent and transfer of that volume from dry vial to dry vial, implying that the
  solution becomes more and more concentrated. The loss bound to
  the incomplete emptying of the content of the vials is proportio-
  nally increased.
- use of a maladjusted diluent.

CONCLUSIONS
_____

Advantages of a centralization in the Pharmacy of preparation
of cytotoxic drugs :
- time economy with personnel of same salary scale : the actual procedure extrapolated to the entire hospital should permit a saving
  of approximately 500 hours per year.
- accuracy of the dosage of the drug really dispensed
- sterility of the preparation
- protection of the preparator and of the work environment
- large decrease of the ward stock of expensive and dangerous
  products.

Disadvantages of a centralization :
- a lack of twenty four hours coverage by the pharmacy : the lack of
  adequate personnel allow this service only from 8,30 a.m. to
  5.30 p.m., during the official opening hours of the Pharmacy.
- a minimal delay of 1 to 2 hours is necessary between the prescription and the administration of the drug.

It is our conviction that the preceding findings are not limited to our hospital but reflect a situation that can be found in many
other institutions.
Not only for the qualitative improvement, but also for the economical
aspect, centralized dispensing of cytotoxic drugs by the hospital Pharmacy offers an interesting solution.

PROGRESS IN THE MANAGEMENT OF HIGH DOSE METHOTREXATE

J. Welsh
Department of Clinical Oncology, Glasgow University.

D. Whitehill
Department of Pharmacy, Robert Gordon's Institute of
Technology, Aberdeen.

T. Habeshaw
Institute of Radiotherapy, Western Infirmary, Glasgow.

P. Billiaert, J.F.B. Stuart, S.B. Kaye, K.C. Calman.
Department of Clinical Oncology, Glasgow University.

Conventionally methotrexate administration is withheld in
patients with impaired renal function or a third space.
The use of the EMIT rapid homogenous enzyme immuno-assay
technique has increased the safety of this drug's use.
We wished to compare the efficacy of a titration technique
incorporating bedside monitoring of MTX by EMIT with that of
a method which involved the calculation of the amount of MTX
required to produce a desired level.
Each method proved equally efficacious. We investigated
the effect of probenicid on the excretion of MTX finding
that the $t_{\frac{1}{2}}$ gamma was delayed and recommend that a patient
receiving these drugs concurrently is closely monitored.
With prudent MTX monitoring no toxicity was achieved in a
patient whose renal function was impaired (creatinine
clearance 30 mls/min.). This patient was given reduced
doses of MTX. In a patient who developed acute renal
failure following MTX chemotherapy, facilities which provided
rapid plasma MTX measurement were invaluable in determining
the amount and duration of folinic acid rescue. In
conclusion MTX must be used with caution and monitoring
facilities should be widely available.

PHARMACOKINETICS OF CYTOSINE ARABINOSIDE IN LEUKEMIC PATIENTS
WITH NORMAL AND IMPAIRED HEPATIC FUNCTIONS. PRELIMINARY RESULTS

C. MONTAGNIER, Ph.D, M.J. FERRER et A. ASTIER, Ph.D.
Toxicology and Pharmacology Laboratory, Pharmaceutical Depar-
ment. C. CORDONNIER, M.D. J.P. VERNANT, M.D. AND H. ROCHANT,M.D.
Hematology Department. H. MONDOR HOSPITAL, 94010 CRETEIL -
France.

I. INTRODUCTION

Cytarabine ara.C is an antimetabolite widely used as an anti-
neoplasic agent in the treatment of acute myeloblastic leukemias. After
phosphorylation to ara.CTP, it acts as a pyrimidine analog via competitive
inhibition with DNA polymerase during the S phase. It is thus a phase-
dependent agent. The elimination of ara.C is primarily metabolic.

A deamination enzyme with selective hepatic location, cytidine
aminohydrolase, transforms ara.C to inactive uracil arabinoside or ara.U,
which is excreted by the kidneys. The degree of hepatic activity is thus
a primary factor in total ara.C clearance in humans.

The kinetics of this molecule have been extensively studied,
although to a lesser extent in leukemia patients. Studies on its behavior
in cases of acute myeloblastic leukemia with hepatic insufficiency are
very limited in number.

We present preliminary results obtained with 10 acute myeloblastic leukemia patients receiving a test dose of 5 mg/kg, or 200 mg/m^2,
with an I.V. bolus injection.

II. MATERIALS AND METHODS

10 patients presenting an acute myeloblastic leukemia were
admitted to the study. 4 had a clearcut hepato-cellular cytolitic insufficiency, shown by an unmistakable alteration of hepatic clinical chemistry parameters (Table 1). Among them, the normal levels of alanine aminotransferase and aspartate aminotransferase were increased 8-10 times.

The following experimental plan was used. After performing an
initial biochemical workup, a control blood sample was taken and a dose of
ara.C (5 mg/kg, I.V. bolus) was administered in less than one minute.Blood
samples were then taken at 5, 10, 15, 30, 60, 120 and 240 minutes in hepa-
rinized tubes containing 10 umol of tetrahydrouidine (THU), a specific
inhibitor of cytidine deaminase.

Blood was immediately centrifuged at the patients' bedside and plasmas were stored in ice. Assays were performed within 15 minutes with a specific inverted phase HPLC method, derived from that of Breithaupt and al (2). This method led to the simultaneous assay of ara.C and ara.U with a sensitivity of 0.1 ug/ml. This plan was approved by the Medical Ethics Committee of the Mondor Hospital.

III. RESULTS

The kinetic curves, concentration as a function of time, are shown in fig.1 as means ± standard deviations. The squares/solid lines represent ara.C concentrations and the triangles/dotted lines those of ara.U.

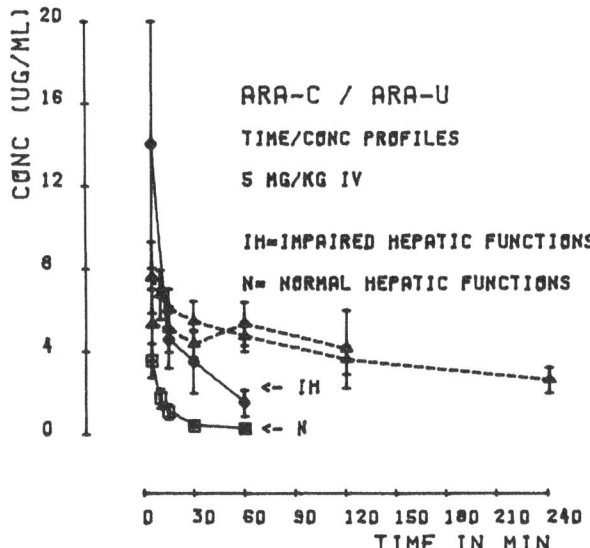

Ara.C disappears rapidly according to a two compartment kinetic model. It may be seen that the ara.A concentrations are statistically greater (p<0.01) in the hepatic insufficiency patients, in spite of a greater variability in the experimental points. The differences for ara.U, on the other hand are not or only slightly significant.

The primary pharmacokinetic parameters obtained for ara.C are shown in Table 2, after computer-assisted filtering. The results indicate a high inter- patient variability for t 1/2 of distribution, t 1/2 of elimination, distribution volume and total clearance.

This finding, as well as mean results calculated for normal subjects, is in good agreement with published data (Baguley et al).

(1) obtained with same type of patient.

Although the differences in t 1/2 values do not appear to be significant, V_D and clearance are statistically decreased in the cytolysis patients.

The ara.U concentration becomes maximal within 5 min of injection, particularly evident in normal subjects. The ara.U/ara.C concentration ratio is greater than two. This had been previously observed by Wan et al, reflecting the considerable first pass effect with this molecule (tab.3). On the other hand, it is interesting to note that the ara.U concentrations at 5 min are much greater than those of ara.C at 5 min. The ara.U/ara.C ratio becomes inverted to a highly significant extent, decreasing from 2.32 to 0.32. Similarly the extrapoled areas under curves show a clear increase ($p < 0.01$) in ara.C in cytolysis patients. The AUC for ara.U/ara.C, very high in normal subjects at 35.1 ± 1.9 ($p < 0.001$) (tab.4). decreases drastically in hepatic insufficiency patients to 5.3 ± 1.9.

IV. DISCUSSION

In the present series, hepatic cytolysis led to a considerable decrease of total ara.C clearance, shown by the inversion of the ara.U/ ara.C ratio, and thus to increased concentrations of ara.C available in the blood.

In hepatic insufficiency patients, the ara.U/ara.C ratio was inverted and V_D decreased drastically from 3.2 1/kg to 0.53 1/kg. This apparently reflects a limitation of the drug distribution in the organism. The clear change in the constants K_{12} and K_{21} argue in favor of this hypothesis. It does not seem that a modification of metabolism is responsible in hepatic insufficiency cases.

Thus :

- metabolism to ara.U is unchanged (AUC of ara.U), since it is the same in both groups;
- there is no reason to believe that there is an amplification of extra-hepatic metabolism. Dédrick et al (2) showed that deaminase activity was primarily hepatic and only very slightly secondarily renal. Extensive plasma deamination may be excluded. A study performed in vitro with whole blood from 6 patients with normal hepatic function demonstrated a very slow deamination (t 1/2 = 180 min);

- a slight decrease of renal excretion of ara.C ($<$10%) cannot
explain the considerable increase of the ara.C concentration
in the blood compartment.

V. CONCLUSION

The present results are interpreted in terms of a limited
extra-blood compartment distribution of ara.C. This results in a decreased efficiency for these patients to distribute the drug to deeper
compartments, e.g. bone marrow target cells, and so to a decreased
clinical efficacy.

This hypothesis is consistent with the highler relapse frequency
observed in patients with clear hepatic dysfunction.

Table 2

NAME	T 1/2 α (min)	T 1/2 β (min)	VD (1/kg)	Cl (ml/min)
Normal hepatic functions				
BEN...	3.1	15.3	2.84	6713
JOU...	8.2	114.4	6.61	2001
URB...	3.4	14.2	0.99	3870
PIA...	2.5	77.9	4.32	2576
FAS...	1.4	22.3	5.39	2100
CHA...	2.5	16.8	1.79	5261
MEAN	3.5	26.8	3.65	3753
± SE	1.4	10.3	0.88	779
Impaired hepatic functions				
ROE...	3.73	20.6	0.44	870
GAG...	1.48	39.7	0.21	203
ACH...*	-	20.8	0.61	1036
LAR...*	-	15.2	0.77	1820
MEAN	-	24.1	0.51	982
± SE	-	5.4	0.12	271

* Monocompartimental NS p$<$0.05   p$<$0.05

Table 3

| NAME | CONCENTRATION at T+5 min(ug/ml) | | Ratio |
	ara.U	ara.C	ara.U/ara.C
Normal hepatic functions			
CHA...	4.42	3.25	1.37
BEN...	5.97	1.77	3.37
JOU...	6.6	3.0	2.20
URB...	14.3	6.71	2.13
PIA...	6.28	2.95	2.13
FAS...	7.96	3.59	2.22
MEAN	7.58	3.54	2.23
SE	1.42	0.68	0.26
Impaired hepatic functions			
ROE...	8.92	20.8	0.43
GAG...	3.04	32.7	0.08
ACH...	1.6	6.87	0.23
LAR...	12	17.6	0.68
MEAN	6.39	19.49	0.36
± SE	2.42	5.31	0.12
	NS	$p < 0.01$	$p < 0.001$

Table 4

NAME	AUC — Ara.C	Ug/ml/min Ara.U	Ratio Ara.U/Ara.C
Normal hepatic functions			
CHA...	66.5	1282	19.3
BEN...	27.3	1860	68.1
JOU...	81.4	784	9.6
PIA...	90.8	1737	19.3
FAS...	27.6	1221	44.2
MEAN	57.9	1595.8	35.1
± SE	10.9	271.8	9.2
Impaired hepatic functions			
ROE...	205	579	2.83
GAG...	688	2697	3.92
ACH...	241	-	-
LAR...	113	1034	9.15
MEAN	331.7	1437.1	5.3
± SE	128.3	643.7	1.95
	$p < 0.01$	NS	$p < 0.01$

1 - BAGULEY B.C. and FALKENBROUG E.M., (1971) plasma half-life of cytosine
    arabinoside in patients treated for acute myeloblastie leukemia,
    cancer chemother., Rep., $\underline{55}$, 291-298.

2 - BREITHAUPT H. and SCHICK J.C., 1981, determination of cytarabine
    and uracil arabinoside in human plasma and cerebrospinal fluid by
    high performance liquid chromatography. J. of chromatogr., Biomed
    appl., $\underline{225}$, 99-106.

3 - DEDRICK R.L., FORRESTER D.D., CANNON J.N., EL DAREER S.M. and
    MELLETT L.B., (1973), Pharmacokinetic of 1- -D. Arabinosifuronosyl-
    cytosine (ara.C). Deamination in Several Species, Biochem. Pharmacol.
    $\underline{22}$, 2405-2417.

THE   OPERATION   OF   A   THERAPEUTIC   TEAM   IN   DERMATOLOGY

A. Dooms-Goossens
Contact Dermatitis Unit, Department of Dermatology,
University Hospital, B-3000 Leuven, Belgium

M. Dooms,
Pharmacy Department,
University Hospital, B-3000 Leuven, Belgium

J. Durgin
Director of Clinical Pharmacy Programs,
St. John's University, Jamaica, New York, 11439

R. Roelandts
Photobiology Unit, Department of Dermatology,
University Hospital, B-3000 Leuven, Belgium

H. Degreef
Professor of Dermatology,
University Hospital,B-3000 Leuven, Belgium

Abstract. This report concerns the concept of the therapeutic team and the respective contributions and responsibilities of pharmacists, nurses, and physicians to the
planning and implementation of drug treatment regimes. The
experience of a health care team approach of two pharmacists and two physicians to drug treatment in dermatology
is reported. The emphasis is placed on the clinical pharmacy services in the pharmacy department as well as in the
dermatology department: dispensing pharmaceuticals, compounding liquid and semi-liquid dosage forms, documenting
professional activities, prescribing drugs, direct patient
involvement, education, and consultation. Four clinical
cases--acne, psoriasis, contact dermatitis, and vitiligo--
are presented that involved discussion between dermatologists and pharmacists.

INTRODUCTION

The theme of the 11th European Symposium on Clinical Phar-
macy--the concept of the therapeutic team and the contribution and
responsibilities of pharmacists, nurses, and physicians in planning
and implementing drug treatment regimes--is both important and uni-
versal.

This theme is one that has allowed us to progress to the
point where we can begin to address the real issues at stake: the
contribution of each discipline and the competencies and skills required of each team member. We believe that this Symposium has also

provided the occasion for attitudes, feelings, and professional concerns to emerge and to be brought into the open for further consideration, debate, and even challenge.

As health-care professionals, we have at least one thing in
common: the concern for the ultimate good of the patient. This will
be accomplished not by looking at each other and asking why but by
looking at the patient, together, and asking how. How we can each,
with the knowledge, skills, and concerns of our own discipline contribute to and implement the service of the other professionals.

Prof. Dr. Bogaert mentioned earlier in this symposium that
our contribution will depend on:

1. where we practice

2. the clinical competency levels that are possessed by the various members of the health care team and

3. the clinical competency skills that we, as pharmacists, have
   assiduously acquired and are able to apply.

Regarding the where, the problems referred to in this symposium are no
different from the problems in the U.S, where there is a clinical
pharmacy bell curve and most of the writing is being done by the avant
garde! We do not want to contradict an earlier speaker who indicated
that 25% of the pharmacists in the U.S. practice so-called "clinical
pharmacy" but, from the expérience in the Greater New York City area,
we would say it is closer to 2%. Therefore, it is important for all
of us to examine the efforts of those who have made the therapeutic
team not a slogan but a reality.

There is such a team at the University Hospital in Leuven, Belgium, and it has been functioning for six years now. The specific
therapeutic concern of this team is a very significant one: dermatology. The signs here are evident: the erythemas, wheals, blisters,
and boils. And the symptoms are persistent: itching, burning, pain,
and annoyance. These patients need help. Most of them are referrals,
people who have sought help previously in vain. In Leuven, an expert
panel of physicians and pharmacists works in concert in making the
diagnoses, devising the treatment plans, coordinating the research,
and supervising the product formulation for the alleviation of dermal
pathologies.

The panel consists of Prof. Dr. Degreef, Director of Dermatology,
Dr. Rik Roelandts, a dermatologist with a strong research interest,

Dr. An Dooms-Goossens, a pharmacist directly involved in patient care, and Marc Dooms, a pharmacist who has developed specialized skills in the formulation of dermatological preparations.

CLINICAL PHARMACY SERVICES IN DERMATOLOGY

At their meeting in Minnesota in 1981, the Committee on Clinical Pharmacy as a Specialty defined clinical pharmacy as follows:

> Clinical Pharmacy is a health-science specialty whose responsibility it is to assure the safe and appropriate use of drugs in patients through the application of specialized knowledge and functions in patient care and which necessitates specialized education and/or structured training. It requires use of judgment in the collection and interpretation of data, patient-specific involvement and direct interprofessional interaction.

Five years of experience in a dermatology unit has shown us that a pharmacist can become an active participant on the patient-care team and has a unique contribution to be made on the basis of his or her knowledge in the field of drug use and, here, the safe and appropriate use of drugs on the human skin. In the literature, however, we have found little on the role of the clinical pharmacist in dermatology (Bond 1975).

In the Pharmacy Department, we deal with dermatology in three ways: by dispensing pharmaceuticals, by compounding liquid and semi-solid dosage forms, and by documenting professional activities. These three classic functions are interpreted in the broadest sense. We not only dispense pharmaceuticals marketed in Belgium, we also order from other countries those that are not or not yet marketed here, such as TIGASON (etrinate 25 mg) from Roche, Hertfordshire, England, MELADININE solution (methoxsalen) from Promedica, Paris, France, and CG-217 (thalidomide 100 mg) from Grünenthal, Stolberg, Germany. We compound the regularly prescribed formulas and also, if necessary, formulations before they come on the market such as benzoylperoxide 5% and 10% cream, clindamycin 1% lotion, aluminum trichloride 20% alcoholic lotion, Monsels solution, dihydroxyaceton lotions, and anthralin anhydrous water washable ointment. A considerable amount of effort is also put into designing formulas for particular patients, such as a lanolin-free w/o cream for lanolin-sensitive patients.

Concerning drug information, we deal with questions concerning the price, package size, and reimbursement of dermatologicals
as well as dermal toxicity and comparative pharmacological activity.
The Pharmacy Department also contributes to the up-dating of the Product File of our CODEX system, a computer readable data base used to
assist in the diagnosis and treatment of contact dermatitis patients.
This file contains the complete composition (active and non-active
ingredients alike) of all the pharmaceutical products in Belgium that
are used in contact with the skin and the mucous membranes (Dooms-
Goossens et al. 1980).

Finally, we have worked out a chemical method for monitoring concentrations of methoxsalen in patients with psoriatic lesions.
This procedure is now routine in the Toxicology Laboratory (Roelandts
et al. 1981a).

In the Dermatology Department, we deal with special pharmaceutical functions: prescribing drugs, direct patient involvement,
education, and consultation.

When a patient suspected of a contact dermatitis reaction
comes to the clinic, he is sent to the Contact Dermatitis Unit where
he is seen by a team of three medical professionals: a pharmacist, a
resident in dermatology, and a laboratory technician. After the anamnesis is taken, patch testing is performed with the international
standard series and with other suspected agents. When a patient re-
acts positively to a certain ingredient, its relevance is checked in
the Product File. This computer readable file is available on-line
with a CRT display screen and on microfilm at the Contact Dermatitis
Unit. After diagnosis, the patient is given a computer print-out of
all of the pharmaceutical products containing the specific allergens,
and the anamnesis is entered into the computer for statistical analysis.

DISCUSSION OF CLINICAL CASES

1. ACNE

Acne is a skin disease of the pilosebaceous follicle. The
primary lesion involves an inflammation of this follicule resulting in
a variety of lesions: comedones, cysts, papules, pustules, and nodules.

Benzoylperoxide, a topical antibacterial agent with comedo-
lytic properties, is used in the treatment of this disease. On the
occasion of its use in the topical therapy of leg ulcers as 20% lotion
(Colman & Roenigk 1978), benzoylperoxide was found to be an important
skin sensitizer. When used in the proper concentrations, however, its
overall cutaneous safety has been demonstrated for acne patients (Cunliffe & Burke 1982).

Several antibiotics such as clindamycin and erythromycin
have been used successfully in the topical treatment of acne. Only
antibiotics with a low sensitization potential should be used for such
treatment because there is always the danger that the patient will
become sensitized to ingredients that he may be in urgent need of
should he contract a severe infection.

2. Psoriasis

Psoriasis is one of the most common skin disorders, about
2% to 3% of the population being affected. Although the sites of
predilection are the elbows and knees, the entire body can be affected. Not so long ago, severe cases of psoriasis required hospit-
alization, but in recent years, even these patients can be treated on
an outpatient basis thanks to photochemotherapy (PUVA therapy). This
treatment consists of combining the administration of 8-methoxypsora-
len (8-MOP) with long-wave UV irradiation. The patient takes a constant dose of 8-MOP orally in function of his body weight. Two hours
later, when the 8-MOP serum level is expected to be maximized, the
patient receives whole body ultraviolet irradiation using a special
light box with the emission spectrum in the UV-A range. This is
usually done three times a week until the condition clears up completely. An average of 21 irradiations are required (7 weeks). A
major step in optimizing PUVA therapy is the standardization of the
8-MOP serum levels (Roelandts et al. 1981b). It is important that the
time of the UV-A irradiation coincides with the maximum 8-MOP serum
level and that this level is as high as possible. Many intraindi-
vidual and interindividual variations have been reported: differences
in absorption rates, metabolism, and a first-pass effect in the liver
can account for interindividual 8-MOP serum level variation. Day-to-
day variations can also occur in the same individual. We have shown
that there is a dietary influence and that the dietary conditions in

which the 8-MOP is taken have to be standardized (Roelandts et al. 1981a). In addition, the drug form is of critical importance because the particle size and the crystal form of the 8-MOP, its presentation form, and the way this presentation form is made can significantly influence the 8-MOP serum levels (Van Boven et al., 1982). Therefore, we are now conducting trials with different forms of 8-MOP in collaboration with our School of Pharmacy.

3. Contact Dermatitis

Allergic contact dermatitis results from the exposure of sensitized individuals to contact allergens or sensitizers. In the acute phase, an allergic contact dermatitis is characterized by redness, edema, papules, vesiculation, weeping, and crusting and is accompanied by pruritis. If it becomes chronic, the skin may become thickened, lichenified, fissured, and pigmented. The diagnosis of a contact dermatitis reaction is confirmed by patch testing, the materials and methods of which have been standardized by the International Contact Dermatitis Research Group (Fregert 1981).

Pharmaceutical products may contain such sensitizers. A multi-center study conducted in Belgium (Dooms-Goossens 1982) revealed the following substances to be the ten most sensitizing ingredients in topical pharmaceuticals:

1. Wool alcohols
2. Neomycin
3. Anorganic mercury compounds
4. Benzocaine
5, Sulphanilamide
6. Balsam of Peru
7. Ethylenediamine hydrochloride
8. Wood tar
9. Thiomersal
10. Cetyl alcohol

The only therapy for these patients is the avoidance of their specific allergens. Fortunately, modern medicine does not need these sensitizers or has found safer alternatives for them. Substances such as balsam of Peru have negligible pharmacological activity, and other allergens can easily be replaced by less sensitizing ingredients with comparable activity. For example, benzocaine can be replaced by lidocaine, neomycin by polymyxin and mercurial antiseptics by povidone iodine.

4. Vitiligo

Vitiligo is a disease whereby, for unknown reasons, the melanocytes become inactive and disappear from the epidermis. Thus, irregular depigmentations of the skin occur that are very disturbing esthetically especially in the dark complexions. Several treatments have been introduced such as PUVA and the local application of corticosteroids and psoralens, but the results have been erratic and disappointing. Generally all that can be done for this skin disease is to mask the lesions with dihydroxyaceton lotions.

CONCLUSION

As we bring this panel discussion to a close, we hope many of us will see opportunities to "go and do likewise".

The allusions to our need for more people, more money, and more equipment may be more fancy than fact. But we do need more conviction, courage, competency, and willingness to face a challenge. The Dermatology Team at the Leuven University Hospital could well be an example to follow. What we have accomplished in dermatology could well be applicable in pediatrics, psychiatry, coronary care, emergency services, and all the other therapeutic specialties where there is an obvious need and where a willing to acquire the necessary competence and to contribute to patient care in a purposeful and meaningful way.

FORMULATIONS CITED

1. Benzoylperoxide cream (Pace 1968)

   Benzoylperoxide 5% or 10%

   Chloroform 3.5% or 7%

   Cetyl alcohol 15 g

   White beeswax 1 g

   Propylene glycol 10 g

   Sodium lauryl sulphate 2 g

   Water ad 100 g

2. Clindamycin 1% lotion

   Clindamycin phosphate 1%

   Isopropyl alcohol 50 g

   Sodium hydroxide solution 10% to adjust pH = 5.5

   Water ad 100 g

3. Aluminum trichloride 20% alcoholic lotion (Scholes et al. 1978)

   Aluminum chloride hexahydrate 20%

   Absolute alcohol

4. Monsels solution (Martin and Cook 1956)

   Ferrous sulphate 1045 g

   Sulphate acid 55 ml

   Nitric acid q.s.

   Purified water ad 100 ml

5. Dihydroxyaceton lotion

   Dihydroxyaceton 4 to 12 g

   Aceton 1 to 3 g

   Alcohol 50 g

   Water ad 100 g

6. Anthralin anhydrous water washable ointment

   Anthralin 0.5% to 3%

   Emulsifying wax 30 g

   Hard paraffin 20 g

   White soft paraffin ad 100 g

7. Lanolin-free w/o cream

   White soft paraffin 5 g

   Arlacel C 83 6 g

   Water ad 100 g

REFERENCES

Bond, C.A. (1975).   Skin diseases.   In Clinical Pharmacy and Therapeu-
    tics, eds. Eric T. Herfindal & Joseph L. Hirschman, pp.
    441-457. Baltimore: Williams and Wilkins Company.
Colman, G.J. & Roenigk, H.H. (1978). Topical therapy of leg ulcers with
    20 percent benzoyl peroxide lotion. Cutis, 11, 491-494.
Committee Pursuing Specialty Recognition for Clinical Pharmacy Holds
    Meeting (1982). Am. J. Hosp. Pharm.,39, 376.
Cunliffe, W.J. & Burke, B. (1982). Benzoyl peroxide: lack of sensitiza-
    tion. Acta Dermatol. 62, 458-459.
Dooms-Goossens, A., Degreef, H., Drieghe, J. & Dooms, M. (1980). Compu-
    puter assisted monitoring of contact dermatitis patients.
    Contact Dermatitis, 6, 123-127.
Dooms-Goossens, A. (1982). Allergic contact dermatitis to ingredients
    used intopically applied pharmaceutical products and cos-
    metics. Unpublished doctoral thesis. Katholieke Universi-
    teit Leuven, Leuven, Belgium.
Fregert, S. (1981). Manual of Contact Dermatitis. 2nd edition. Copen-
    hagen: Munksgaard.
Martin, E.W. & Cook, E.F. (1956). Ferric subsulfate solution N.F. In
    Remington's Practice of Pharmacy, pp. 576-577. Easton,
    Pennsylvania: The Mack Publishing Company.
Pace, W.E. (1965). A benzoyl peroxide-sulfer cream for acne vulgaris.
    Canad. Med. Ass. J., 93, 252-254.
Roelandts, R., Van Boven, M., Deheyn, T., Vander Stichele, G., Degreef,
    H. & Daenens, P. (1981a). Dietary influences on 8-MOP
    plasma levels in PUVA patients with psoriasis. Br. J. Der-
    matol., 105, 569-572.
Roelandts, R., Van Boven, M., & Adriaens, P. (1981b). Methoxsalen serum
    serum level variations in psoralen and ultraviolet-A (PUVA)
    therapy. Arch. Dermatol., 117, 758.
Scholes, K.J., Crow, K.D., Ellis, J.P., Harman, R.R. & Saihan E.M.
    (1978). Axillary hyperhidrosis treated with alcoholic solu-
    tion of aluminium chloride hexahydrate. Br. Med. J., 2, 84-
    85.
Van Boven, M., Roelandts, R., Adriaens, P., Daenens, P. & Degreef, H.
    (1982). Standardizing 8-MOP plasma profiles by using an
    emulsion form. Arch. Dermatol. (in press).

TEAM TREATMENT OF EPILEPSY

Fred Schobben
Pharmacy of the University Hospital, Utrecht,
the Netherlands

Eppo van der Kleijn
Dpt. Clinical Pharmacy, St. Radboud Hospital, Nijmegen
the Netherlands

MULTIDISCIPLINARY APPROACHES

Care for patients with epilepsy may offer medical, psychosocial and educational or occupational problems. Optimal help requires
co-ordinated efforts by several disciplines. Specialised epilepsy clinics
held by teams including neurologists and social workers appear to be
beneficial to the patients well-being (Cereghino and Cole 1971, Smits et
al. 1976). Severe cases may be admitted to specialised epilepsy centers
with advanced technical possibilities and expert knowledge. However many
patients with epilepsy live in other institutions, e.g. those for the
mentally retarded. Here, co-ordinated approach by several disciplines is
often lacking. The appointment of a nurse specialist, charged with care
for the epileptics, can effectively overcome this problem (O'Neill et al.
1977).

Experts with pharmacological background have seldom been included in treatment teams. The Milano collaborative group for studies on
epilepsy (1977) was probably the first example. Four pharmacologists, one
chemist, one social worker and eight neurologists met monthly to discuss
general problems and 60 "difficult" patients in particular. After a critical phase, during which pessimism dominated, a positive co-operation
evolved. A preliminary evaluation revealed a reduction of drug treatment
and improved control of epilepsy at the same time.

TEAM PROJECT IN INSTITUTIONALISED PATIENTS

Since 1976 142 patients with epilepsy living in an institution for the mentally retarded were treated by a team consisting of
several general practitioners, two psychologists, a secretary and two
external consultants: a neurologist and a pharmacist. The latter acted
as co-ordinator. For each patient a balance was pursued between minimum
seizures, minimum drug treatment and optimal functioning and well-being.

Treatment was adapted following strict guidelines (Schobben 1979). All
decisions were taken by consensus of the team.

Although the prognosis of epilepsy was poor in many patients, drug treatment could be simplified markedly during the first two years. Only after
three years a satisfactory condition was reached in half of the patients.
It took another 3 years to reach ultimate optimal treatment in about the
same group. Comparison of the last two years with the initial period
shows a marked reduction of seizure frequency (table 1). At the same time
the number of drugs per patient had been reduced: Initially most patients
were treated with 2-4 anti-epileptic drugs. Now 50% of all treated
patients has monotherapy. In 14% all anti-epileptic drugs have been withdrawn. Probably as a consequence, the alertness and behaviour of many
patients improved, according to subjective impressions.

Many efforts have been made to reach the indicated results.
The team met for one afternoon a week for at least three years. A large
number of people were involved in continuously monitoring these patients.
Participation of attendants of the patients in team discussions appeared
to be fruitful for optimal co-operation and adequate information. A
centralised administration of all data on the individual patients appears
to add to the efficiency of the team meetings. Graphical recording of
drug dosages, plasma concentrations and seizures was of invaluable help
in difficult cases. Anti-epileptic drug plasma level analyses dropped
from average 5 per patient per year below one per year. Since the pharmacist-co-ordinator has left the team after 3½ years the number of drug
analyses rose again, although the number of changes of drug treatment
continued to decrease. From this period the need for strict co-ordination

Table 1. Change of seizure frequency during the project

initial condition	satisfactory control	unsatisfactory control
100% reduction	11	9
remained seizure free	20	–
over 50% reduction	2	19
unchanged	11	36
over 50% increase	9	5
only occasional seizures	9	–
	(n = 62)	(n = 69)

became evident. During the project the knowledge on epilepsy of all
participants has greatly increased. Consultant specialists felt more
productive in the team than as individual advisers in isolated cases.
Unfortunately no sufficient means were available for objective or quantitative evaluation of changes in functioning and well-being of the
patients.

ROLE OF PHARMACIST

For meaningful interpretation of drug plasma levels and the
maximum profit in individual dosing, expertise in pharmacokinetics is a
prerequisite. If this is realised by a pharmacist he may make use of his
other abilities in the systematic treatment of epilepsy. Although this
seems contradictory in private practice, an institutional pharmacist
appears to exert the major insistance on reduction of drug use and limitation of plasma level analyses. Of course any other of the team members
may act as co-ordinator for the activities and services. However, monitoring and guarding of the treatment protocol, once it has been agreed
upon, will have to be executed by a person with unbiased judgement.
Having no direct competence in relation to the patients, the pharmacist
is a good candidate if not the best. Recording of individual drug prescriptions and plasma level analyses belongs to the pharmacist's regular
tasks. Addition of clinical parameters like seizure frequency, EEG results and behavioural scores to his files is basically only a minor step.
Therefore full patient documentation is centralised preferably under
supervision of the pharmacist-co-ordinator.

In practice, the role of the pharmacist is only valuable when
he is an integral part of the joint approach of several disciplines.

ACKNOWLEDGEMENTS

The authors wish to thank the team-neurologist, H.M. Vingerhoets, Dpt. Neurology, St. Radboud Hospital, Nijmegen and all staff members of the institute for the mentally retarded "Huize Boldershof",
Druten, the Netherlands, for their indispensable and stimulating
co-operation in the project described here.

REFERENCES
Cereghino, J.J. and Cole, C.H. (1971) A multidisciplinary approach to
services for the epileptic. HSMHA Health Reports 86, 355-371.

Milano collaborative group for studies on epilepsy (1977) Long-term
          intensive monitoring in the difficult patient. Preliminary
          results of 16 months of observations - usefullness and
          limitations. In: Gardner-Thorpe, C., Janz, D., Meinardi,H.
          and Pippenger, C.E., Eds. Anti-epileptic drug monitoring,
          Pitman Medical, Kent, England, 197-213.
O'Neill, B.O., Ladon, B., Harris, L.M., Riley, H.L. and Dreifuss, F.E.
          (1977) A comprehensive, interdisciplinary approach to the
          care of the institutionalised person with epilepsy.
          Epilepsia 18, 243-250.
Schobben, A.F.A.M. (1979) Pharmacokinetics and therapeutics in epilepsy.
          Thesis, Catholic University, Nijmegen, the Netherlands.
Smits, H., Bakker, H.S.M. and Veenhof, A. (1976) Extramurale aktiviteit
          in het kader van epilepsiebestrijding. Tijdschr. Soc.
          Geneeskunde 54, 106-116.

PRACTICES OF THE THERAPEUTIC TEAM IN EPILEPSY

P. Loiseau
Clinique Neurologique, Hôpital Pellegrin, 33076 Bordeaux Cedex, France

INTRODUCTION
The standpoint of a physician will be illustrated by the
experience of the department of neurology of the University of Bordeaux.
Epileptics attend   this department either as out-patients or as in-
patients.

OUT-PATIENTS

1 Previously-untreated patients

The therapeutic team is simple : practitioner and a specialist.
In most cases general practitioners do not see current epileptic patients
and are not very familiar with antiepileptic therapy. The specialist must
explain why to choose a drug according to the clinical form of epilepsy,
how to determine the daily drug dose and the dosage regimen. He has also
to explain that a one-drug treatment is more convenient than polypharmacy.
The aim and the long duration of therapy have to be explained to the
patient.

2 Previously-treated patients

1°. If the patient is seizure-free and demonstrates no side
effect of drug, the specialist's role is to avoid unnecessary plasma level
measurements or, if the determination is already done, to avoid a rise of
the daily dose because of too low a plasma level. Indeed about one-third
of epileptics may be controlled with low doses and plasma levels below the
usually recommended range. However patients and physicians are more
confident in lab. examination than in clinical evidence and it is very
difficult to explain that plasma levels are not a panacea.

2°. In case of persistent seizures or in patients controlled
but with clinical signs of overdosage, routine therapeutic drug monitoring
is mandatory. This monitoring value is now well documented. The kinetics
of a drug are subject to wide interindividual variations. Measurements of

plasma concentration yields a much better correlation with the patient's
clinical status than does total daily drug dosage. However optimizing drug
therapy with plasma level monitoring needs a careful analysis of plasma
levels.Clinical and lab.information has to be carefully analysed.
A blood level is only a number. This number results from many factors :
the drug's own kinetics, for instance its absorption, distribution,
metabolism and excretion in a particular individual in a given physiological status. The age and the weight of the patient, his compliance, the
sampling time, the steady-state, and co-medication are discussed by the
pharmacist and the physician.
Plasma levels will allow to individualize drug therapy and to modify its
daily dosage in order to achieve a level in the therapeutic range. In this
therapeutic range the drug is supposed to have a maximum of efficacy and a
minimum of side-effects for the majority of patients. However "there is no
such thing as a therapeutic range applicable to all patients, unless it be
from just above zero to the top of the optimum range" (Reynolds 1980). It
is important to note that some patient do not demonstrate any clinically
toxic sign with plasma levels which in most patients are correlated with
toxic signs. In these cases serum concentration is not nearly as important
as the clinical judgement.

IN-PATIENTS

1 *Previously-untreated patients*
   In a ward the patient meets many persons and usually asks the
same questions to several persons. They must be able to give homogenous
replies. These interrogations of course concern the evolution and prognosis
of epilepsy and drug therapy. Moreover if seizures occur, they will not
have the same witness. A high level of information is necessary for the
therapeutic team. It is given at two different levels. Each physician
(specialist, assistants, residents), and each nurse in the ward must have
a general education about epileptic seizures and antiepileptic drugs,
through lectures, films and informal meetings. Each physician and each
nurse must know, as soon as possible, details of the particular patient
they have to treat. A meeting is held for each individual case. Everyone
explains what he has observed about this patient's behavior and seizures.
Social workers and psychologists are eventually present. The guidelines
for therapy are given to nurses who have to apply it. They are informed,
too, about the possible side effects of the drug : drowsiness, dizziness,
gastro-intestinal troubles, cutaneous rashes, etc... .

2 *Previously-treated epileptics with persistent seizures*

The interface between physicians, pharmacists and nurses here is prominent. If seizures still occur, therapy is modified. The basis is the drug(s) plasma concentration measured as soon as the patient comes into the ward. A systematic sampling is done by a nurse. Previously prescribed therapy is maintained till the result of this measurement is known. Of course a fast determination is very useful. It the dose-response ratio is abnormal, the therapy remains unchanged and further determinations are done to verify if this ratio remains constant. Laboratory data are discussed as they are for out-patients and the daily dosage adjusted to achieve a plasma level in the therapeutic range. In case of persistent seizures despite this optimization of previously-prescribed drug(s) another drug is given. The change is explained to patients first by a physician, then by nurses every time they give tablets to him. Nurses must be aware of its modalities, for instance a progressive shift from a drug to another. Plasma level monitoring is done. The trial is discussed with the pharmacist. Dose and dosage regimen are fixed with the aid of the laboratory data. Loading doses, at least for phenobarbital and phenytoin, are often prescribed, for shortening the patient's stay in the hospital. Pharmacokinetic parameters allow to extrapolate steady-state plasma concentration. Care for sampling, sampling time, amount of blood necessary for assays are explained to nurses by pharmacists. But nothing remains fixed. Our team has existed since 1974. We had in 1981 a serious problem, due to a peak on some chromatograms. Several weeks passed before we found that the plastic material for sampling had been changed, and that the new corks were responsible. Some months later, plasma levels were abnormaly low for patients in steady-state ; we discovered that a new nurse, afraid of blood clotting, used large amounts of anticoagulant. The tubes arrive now directly and ready for use from the laboratory.

3 *Admission for clinical trials*

For therapeutic trials a very careful multidisciplinary approach is mandatory. In a preliminary meeting the aims and the methods are explained. A nurses' consent without ethical problems is necessary. They have to keep in mind how important it is to give the drug and to sample at exact times. Pharmacists contribute to choose the daily dosage which has to be large enough to give valuable plasma levels. To discuss with the whole team the results of these trials is very simulating.

In conclusion, optimization of drug therapy in epilepsy is the result of a rather easy multidisciplinary approach.

INTERDISCIPLINARY APPROACH TO THE TREATMENT OF EPILEPSY

M.J.G. Cremers
Hooge Burch, Centre for mentally handicapped
Spoorlaan 19, 2471 PB Zwammerdam, The Netherlands

Abstract. The advantages of teamwork in the treatment of
epilepsy are as follows:
Teamwork increases the knowledge of the diagnosis of epilepsy,
treatment of choice, side-effects of drugs, stage of development and individual response of the patient.
It promotes the uniform recording of changes in therapy and
their effects with regard to the number and nature of seizures
and the patient's well-being.
It improves interpretation of serum concentrations, interactions and changes in clearance.
It inspires confidence in parents and attendants in the care
with which changes in therapy are carried into effect.

1. Introduction

It is obvious that all factors have to be taken into account
when aiming for optimum therapy of epilepsy. The sedative effect of
various anticonvulsive drugs notably interferes with the development of
the mentally retarded child. But seizures may prevent the mentally
retarded patient from leaving residential care for community care. Hence
the physicians, paediatricians and neurologists involved in the treatment
of epilepsy are important factors in the development of the mentally
retarded.

2. Advantages gained from teamwork

Treatment of epilepsy in the mentally retarded patient should
be based on the following factors: frequency of seizures - type of seizure
-diagnosis of epilepsy - anticonsulsive drug of choice- possible drug
interactions - possible side effects of drugs -patient's stage of development - social and emotional factors relevant to the patient - expectations
of parents and attendants.

Joint consultation held by members of various disciplines is
essential for an overall appraisal of these factors. Interdisciplinary

teamwork ensures that all aspects are fully appreciated. However, it is
not the only advantage of working as a team.

Parents, attendants and in fact physicians are often hesitant
about further optimizing a patient's condition once epileptic symptoms
have stabilized. This accounts for the wait-and-see attitude that is
frequently adopted, leading to potential improvements in therapy not
being carried into effect. The stimulus of a team will pave the way for
a clear decision on whether the prescribed treatment is optimum and
whether any changes are required.

The third advantage of joint action is that the team acts
as a check on whether the proposed changes in therapy are implemented
accordingto the protocol agreed on and whether their effect is evaluated. The acute nature of an epileptic attack prompts swift action. The
protocol as well as the supervision by the team make it easier to cope
with the pressure of the acute condition and will ultimately benefit the
patient.

Moreover, a team dealing with epileptic patients in residential care may act as an incentive to uniform recording of seizures.It
will give a better idea of the long-term effect of changes made in the
patient's medication.

3. Teamwork in practice

As a general physician, I was a member of an epilepsy team
whose aim was to optimize the treatment of a group of mentally retarded
epileptic patients. The team consisted of physicians and psychologists
at the institution and two external consultants: a neurologist and a
pharmacist. A secretary and patients' attendants completed the team.
The team was engaged in:
- choice of therapy. Being a team, it was more knowledgeable and more
motivated by its wish to aim for optimum therapy.

Table 1 number of anti-epileptic drugs per patient

date	01-07-81	01-08-82
none	3	3
1 drug	19	22
2 drugs	27	26
3 drugs	8	7
4 drugs	1	0
average number of drugs per patient:		
total group	1.74	1.64
treated patients only	1.84	1.73

-drug administration. The model for changes in therapy improved and more
allowance was made for drug interactions.

Having taken up a new post in a similar institution that does
not have an epilepsy team, I am now able to compare the two working
situations. To my present post I brought my increased knowledge of the
treatment of epilepsy and the motivation to aim for optimum therapy. Drug
monitoring is available and so is the assistance of a consultant neurologist. However, I have to do without the backing of a consultant pharmacist, the inspiration drawn from discussions on optimum therapy with
fellow team members, the uniform recording of seizures and the supportive knowledge offered by other disciplines.

Of about 180 mentally retarded patients, all of them functioning at severely or profoundly retarded level, 58 suffer from epilepsy
(30%), i.e. 19 female and 39 male patients.

The results of my work as a soloist can be seen by comparing
the anticonvulsive medication on two dates, the intervening period being
13 months (tables 1 and 2).

Comparison of the figures of the two dates against one
another and against the results of other studies shows that there is not
much alteration in anticonvulsive therapy. It may be explained by the fact
that the basic situation as such was reasonably satisfactory. On the other
hand, it may be indicative of the lack of a supportive team when improvements might have been worth pursuing.

Table 2 medication pattern
                        number of patients

date	01-07-81		01-08-82	
phenobarbital	29	50%	23	40%
valproic acid	24	41%	27	47%
phenytoin	18	31%	21	36%
carbamazepine	17	29%	20	34%
clonazepam	2	3%	2	3%
primidone	1	2%	1	2%
diazepam	3	5%	2	3%
ethosuximide	2	3%	1	2%

THE ROLE OF THE CLINICAL PHARMACIST IN THE MONITORING OF AN -
TIEPILEPTIC THERAPY IN CLINICS WITH AMBULANT PATIENTS. OUR EX-
PERIENCE WITH 45 PATIENTS.

MARIA F. ALVAREZ DE TOLEDO
General Practice Pharmacy. Pza. Primo de Rivera. Oviedo. Spain
ROSA MARIA SIMO
Hospital Pharmacy. Ciudad Sanitaria. Oviedo. Spain.

We are going to try to explain our experience of clinical
pharmacy in the monitoring of antiepileptic therapy, as dis--
pensers of the medication and as interpreters of the data on
plasma levels.

The patients that were the material of this study were 45,
whose group characteristics are shown in Table 1, as well as

Table 1 .- Data of the studied population.

TOTAL NUMBER OF PATIENTS STUDIED - 45

SEX: MALE - 20   FEMALE - 25

AGE: (8 - 55 years)

$\ll$ 15 yr - 12

$>$ 15 yr - 33

16 - 35 yr - 24
36 - 55 yr - 8
$>$ 55 yr - 1

THERAPY:	Drug	Patients	%
Monotherapy	CBZ	17	37,8
	DPH	1	2,2
	VA	1	2,2
		19	42,2
Polytherapy	CBZ+PB	10	22,2
	CBZ+PRIM	5	11,2
	CBZ+DPH	1	2,2
	CBZ+VA	1	2,2
	DPH+PB	3	6,7
	VA+CLO	1	2,2
	CBZ+PB+VA	2	4,5
	CBZ+PRIM+DPH	1	2,2
	CBZ+VA+CLO	1	2,2
	CBZ+VA+ETX	1	2,2
		26	57,8

the percentages of monotherapy and polytherapy that were given
to that group (we consider it appropiate to explain that in
this group of epileptic patients Carbamazepine appears as the
most frequent used pharmaceutical product, it does not represent the real average of our therapy in epileptics, on the con
trary it has been conditioned exactly because of the fact that
the analytic determination of this drug was not posible in out
patient clinic of a Neurological Service, where, on the other
hand, the analytical determinations of Diphenylhydantoin and
Phenobarbital, which we think are the most frequently used o-
nes, were possible).

The analytical method employed to know the plasma   levels
of the antiepileptic therapy was the Immune-Enzyme test for
Carbamazepine (CBZ), Primidone (PRIM), and Phenobarbital (PB)
and the Radio-Immune test for Diphenylhydantoin (DPH). These
tests were always carried out in a Laboratory at Barcelona, to
which we mailed the samples (one or two milliliters of serum
of patient).

The moment of taking the patient's sample was carefully -
chosen by us and based on a general criterion for each drug,
following the VAN DER KLEIJN method described in his article
in *Drug Intelligence Clinical Pharmacy* (October, 1980), and
also based on the personal characteristics of the patients.

The results obtained as to pharmacokinetic data of the different analyzed drugs are the following:

As to the patients that only took Carbamazepine (Figure 1)
the relation dose vs. plasma   level could be considered as
hardly having a certain linear relation; we noticed the most
extreme disparities with patients less than 15 years old; with
an average half-life time for this drug of 10, 8 and even 7 -
hours.

Under the patients that took Carbamazepine together with -
another antiepileptic (Figure 2) we were not able to observe
important differences between the association with Phenobarbital or with other drugs. But we did observe frequently, even
with polytherapy, important induction among patients under 15
years of age.

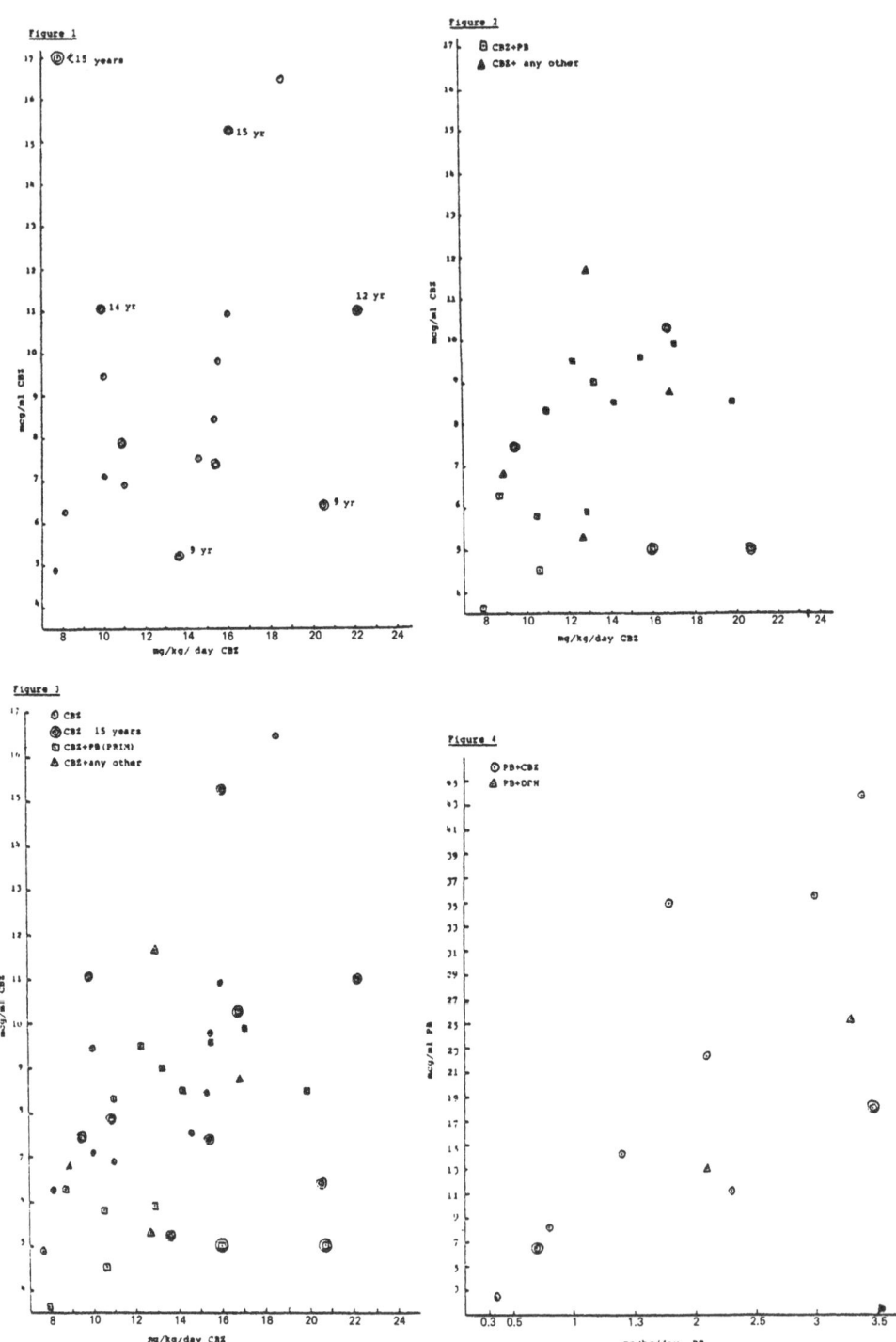

All the same, as we can see in Figure 3, the dispersion of
the results as to the plasma   concentrations of patients in
a steady state   that took Carbamazepine is big. For it is
    easy to prove that for a dose of 16mg/Kg/day, the matic
average plasma concentrations vary between 5 and 16 mcg/ml.
This means that for this drug half-life varies from 7 to
21 hours.

Among the patients that took Phenobarbital the relation dose vs. plasma   level is much more linear, as it has been men
tioned many times in literature and as we can see in Figure 4.

Ultimately the percentage of the toxic and subtherapeutic
levels found in the total   of the analyzed treatments is --
shown on Table 2.

Table 2 .- Percentages of toxic plasma   levels
or subtherapeutic in the studied population.

Monotherapy	Toxic . . . . 4,5 %
	Subtherapeutic . . . . 9,0 %
Polytherapy	Toxic . . . . 4,5 %
	Subtherapeutic . . . 29,0 %

Anyhow we consider that the most interesting features we
should mention HERE and TODAY are not the pharmacokinetic data,
but the problem of the WHAT and HOW of each drug for each individual patient. Our plan was to obtain the best possible
treatment for each single patient, i.e. the most efficient one.
So we tried to:

a) Find out what their therapeutic treatment (drugs, doses, and
dosification pattern) was.

b) Perform extractions in order to determine their plasma levels
at a moment or at the moment most suitable to obtain this
information.

c) Draw possible logical conclusions from the above data.

d) Give the resulting information in the best useful way to the
physician and advise him on many occasions as to modifications
of doses, of frequency and drug use in order to obtain more
appropriate therapeutic results.

Without any doubt the factors to be considered vary with

each drug we studied, so that the information we can offer is
also different; e.g. with Carbamazepine it is important to find
out its average life time in each patient, as this will condition the intervals between each dose; we think it is possible
to calculate them with only   laboratory data. On the other
hand, in the case of Phenobarbital we just inform about the
therapeutic or toxic levels. In the few cases of studies of –
phenytoin we considered it important to perform plasma   level   determinations, where possible, twice, and with different doses.

In Figure 5 a typical sample is shown about our information
to the physician in cases of Carbamazepine. Here the
graph of plasma concentrations during 24 hours is shown,
calculated from the data received from the Laboratory at 11a.m.

Figure 5 .- Graphic representation of the plasmatic levels of Carbamazepine during 24 hours.

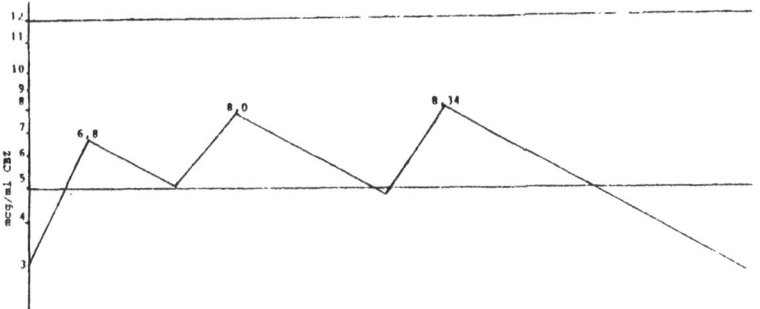

Figure 6 .- Graphic representation of the plasmatic levels of Carbamazepine during 24 hours
          - - - - graphic done with Laboratory data (10 blood samples in 24 hours)
          ___ ___ graphic done with theoretical data after one blood sample at 10 at morning

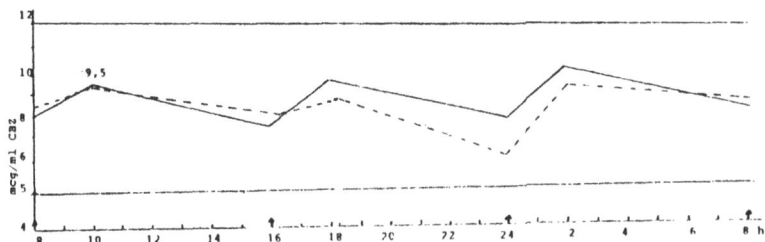

Following VAN DER KLEIJN'S criterion, the sample was extracted
from the patient in the supposed moment of maximum plasma
concentration, after the first intake of the drug.

Figure 6 shows the graph   obtained with laboratory concentrations performed every two hours and the theoretical one we
would have given to the physician with only one extraction.

As a conclusion we think that it belongs to the
clinical pharmacist's functions, to collaborate with the medical team in order to obtain the optimum use of these special
    laboratory data. This function has to be considered from
two sides:

a) As to the patient, to obtain the best and most realistic
treatment.

b) In collaboration with the medical team, to give them
valuable information obtained from the drug history
and the plasma level of the drug.

AN APPROACH TO THE THERAPEUTIC STRATEGY IN RHEUMATOID ARTHRI-
TIS - ADVERSE REACTIONS TO PENICILLAMINE - LIKE DRUGS USED IN
THE TREATMENT OF R.A.

M.H. BROU, J.A.CANAS DA SILVA, E. de PAP and M.VIANA DE QUEI-
RÓS.
Departamentos de Farmácia e Reumatologia, Serviço de Medicina
IV, Hospital Universitário de Santa Maria, Lisboa, PORTUGAL.

We have chosen Rheumatoid Arthritis as the main subject of
our exposition, because it is a disease that enables the therapeutic team
to face many problems during the treatment of the patient; it is neverthe
less highly controlable when correctly managed.

Rheumatoid Arthritis is also a most important social problem,
because of its prevalence (3% in women and 1% in men) and of the conse -
quences in daily activities of the patients.

Finaly it is a chronic disease, presenting problems to be resolved in the medium or long - term, with frequent and serious episodes
requiring urgent care.

Until now R.A. is a disease of unknown aetiology. The fundamen
tal aims of its treatment are:

1 - Relief of pain and inflammation

2 - Maintenance of articular functions

3 - Avoidance of deformities

To attain these fundamental objectives in practice it is neces
sary to have a well prepared therapeutic team able to answer the multiple
needs of the rheumatoid patient.

In this therapeutic team we mention the Rheumatologist, the Or
thopaedist, the Clinical Pharmacist, the Physiotherapist, the Nurse and
the Social Worker.

The treatment of R.A. must be clearly personalized, at the time of the organization of a therapeutic program.

As part of this therapeutic program we have obviously the therapeutic tools and the strategy for the use of these tools, ordered
according to their value for adaptation to each case.

The sucess of the therapeutic program depends greatly on the
correct choice of the tools and the strategy for their use, and the maintenance of an adequate relationship between physician and patient as well

as patient's family. Early diagnosis of the disease is mandatory.

At the base of this therapeutic program there is the correct education of the patient (and his family), reassurance and adequate rest.

The education of the patient must include a brief explanation of the nature of the disease and its chronic and fluctuating character. The physician should show a moderate optimism, avoiding anything which may cause panic or give rise to an exaggerated optimism.

The patient must be correctly informed about the therapeutic program applicable to his case with due regard to his intellectual level. The clinical pharmacist has an important role in explaining the adverse reactions of the drugs and the essential rules to be followed in monito - ring the treatment.

A responsible team should familiarize the patient with the adverse reactions of each drug (without causing apprehension) and be prepa red for an early recognition of these adverse reactions and their correct treatment.

Besides patient's education, the education of his family is ve ry important because of the repercussions of the disease in the family unit. Very often it is also necessary to educate the physician in charge because general practitioners frequently replace all the treatment of RA by the prescription of some other pill which he favours.

Because of the time limitations we will only mention by name the social aspects of the disease, sexual life, compensatory devices and their adaptation in the home and at work, social and professional integration, which are points that the therapeutic team should try to improve positi- vely.

General measures, which include rest and psychological support should be mentioned in a more detailed form.

The time for resting must vary according to the activity of the disease. Thus, in the very active phases of the disease almost comple- te rest is advised, ideally in a hospital, permitting the correct evalua - tion, better understanding of the case and the initiation of the compli- mentary therapeutic measures.

During the more active stages, rest should be daily, not too exaggerated and distributed along the day. At the same time adequate exer- cises should be performed to maintain the articular function.

As for the psychological support its importance can never be exaggerated. Any group that will not be able to maintain a stable, compre-

hensive and adequate relationship with its patients, will not be successful.

In our experience a good psychological outlook is also the
best way to avoid quackery.

Finally, associated diseases (eg: psychologic depression)
should be carefully treated, otherwise they may lead to incomplete trea -
tment.

The drugs used in the treatment of Rheumatoid Arthritis must
be given in a certain order; it is usual to begin the treatment with NSAIDS
(non steroidal anti-inflammatory drugs). If adequate control is not obtained or for by other reasons, one goes on to the second line drugs such as
gold salts, penicillamine, antimalarials and levamisol, which act as immunomodulators.

Corticosteroids and immunosupressors are seldom used; yet, cor
ticosteroids are used by some rheumatologists in low doses (5 to 7.5 mg
prednisolone).

It should be stressed that anti-inflammatory therapy is mainly
symptomatic giving relief only for a short period; this is why the second-
line drugs are of indisputable interest.

Our objective was to evaluate the adverse reactions of gold
salts, penicillamine, and levamisol in the treatment of Rheumatoid Arthritis. The study of their possible relationship with the HLA system of each
patient was also entertained.

Gold salts were introduced in the treatment of Rheumatoid Arthritis about 50 years ago.

D-penicillamine was used for the first time by Walshe in 1955
for Wilsons's disease. Later on, Jaffe reported its interest in Rheumatoid
Arthritis; it has been used also in heavy metal intoxication, in cystinuria, and systemic sclerosis, and in primary biliary cirrhosis.

Levamisol was initially used as an anti-helmintic drug and only in 1974 its immunoregulatory action was used in the treatment of Rheumatoid Arthritis.

Characteristics of the studied population

139 caucasian patients with the diagnosis of Rheumatoid Arthritis according to the criteria of ARA - (American Rheumatism Association)
were evaluated. In this group, 104 were women and 35 were men.

The ages varied between 24 and 72 years, with an average age
of 52.9 years. The duration of the disease oscillated between 3 and 60

years. Besides Rheumatoid Arthritis 23 patients had an associated Sjö - gren's Syndrome.

Seventeen (17) patients had nodules, eighty two (82) had erosive lesions and ninety nine (99) had a seropositive rheumatoid Igm factor.

Patients on immunomodulatory therapy, had classic and defined Rheumatoid Arthritis, for more than 6 months and it has not been possible to control the disease with general measures (rest, non-steroidial anti- inflammatory drugs and physical therapy).

In our Rheumatology Unit we usually prefer a gold salt (aurothio propanol sodio sulfonate) as first choice. We start with 25mg/weekly in the in the first and second administration and then 50 mg/weekly until a total dose of 1.0 g. Later in those patients who responded to the therapy and had no adverse reactions which would lead them to be withdrawn we usually gave a dose of 50 mg every month.

D - penicillamine was used in patients with a history of adverse reactions to gold salts or therapeutic failure and in 25 patients as the initial drug.

The methodology of its use was the administration of 300mg/day during the first and the second month, 600 mg/day during the third and the fourth month and 900 mg/day on the fifth and sixth month.

After this period, patients who responded to the therapy and with no adverse reactions which would oblige one to interrupt the trea - tment, remained with the minimal effective dose.

Levamisol was only used when there was intolerance or lack of therapeutic response to gold salts or D- penicillamine.

Patients with a positive B 27 test were excluded because of the high incidence of side effects to levamisol. The dosage was 150 mg/weekly.

At the begining of the treatment with anyone of these drugs, all the patients were submitted to a clinical and laboratory protocol that in- cluded:

- History and physical examination
- Full blood count: ESR, blood glucose, urea, study of hepatic and renal functions, coagulation test, protein electrophore- sis and detection of rheumatoid factors IgM.
- Control during therapy consisted of the following: for gold salts and d-penicillamine - full blood count, and urine ana- lysis with measurement of proteinuria, weekly, during the first month and every week till the maintenance dose was rea

ched and then every month.

The control with levamisol therapy was a full blood count, 12 hours after   administration.

Before therapy with immunomodulators was initiated the possible interactions between these drugs and other medicaments that the patient was receiving , were considered.

In the following tables we summarise the adverse reactions to gold salts, penicillamine and levamisol.

TABLE I

Adverse reactions to gold salts - 84 patients

Adverse reactions	Patients		Notes	
	nº	%		
Dermatitis	16	16/84 19	withdraw	14
Stomatitis	8	6/84 9.5	"	5
Nephropathy (proteinuria)	9	9/84 10.6	"	5
Haematology (Thrombocytopenia leucopenia)	3	3/84 3.5	"	2
Total Number of adverse reactions	36	36/84 42.8	(31%)	26

TABLE II

Adverse reactions to D-penicillamine - 41 patients

Adverse reactions	Patients		Notes	
	nº	%		
Stomatitis	3	3/41	7.3	withdrawn 1
Nephropathy	5	5/41	12.2	" 1
(proteinuria)				
Dermatitis	3	3/41	7.3	
Myasthenia	1	1/41	2.4	" 2
Haematology	4	4/41	10	" 3
(agranulocytosis)				
(leucopenia)				
(thrombocytosis)				
loss of taste	1	1/41	2.4	
Total number of adverse reactions	19	17/41	41.6	(14,6%) 6

TABLE III

Adverse reactions to levamisol   - 14 patients

Adverse reactions	Patients		Notes	
	nº	%		
Influenza - like syndrome	3	3/14	21.4	withdrawn 2
Weight gain (more than 10Kg)	1	1/14	7.1	" 1
Total number of adverse reactions	4	4/14	28.5	(21,4%) 3

The patients who received immunomodulators were submitted to type tests HLA A,B, C and DR. A correlation was found between some markers and adverse reactions.

An increase of occurence of adverse reactions was verified in the carriers of A_2. Of the thirty four (34) patients with adverse reactions to gold, thirteen (13) patients were carriers of A_2, while of the fifty three (53) patients without adverse reactions only six (6) patients had A_2. However this correlation is not statistically significant.

On the other hand, the correlation between antigen DR 3 and the occurence of proteinuria induced by gold salts was studied, the result being statistically significant (p $<$0,001).

For this reason, we have widened our study with the type test to a total number of one hundred fifty (150) patients, being treated with gold salts.

Of these 150 patients, 18 developed proteinuria. Of the 132 without proteinuria, 39 (29,5%) were carriers of antigen DR 3 and 93 (70,5%) were not. Of the 18 patients with proteinuria, 11 (61,1%) were carriers of antigen and 7 (38,9%) were not.

TABLE IV

Correlation between antigen DR 3 and proteinuria induced by gold salts

DR 3	Proteinuria	
	Present - 18	Absent - 132
Present 50	11 (61,1%)	39 (29,5%)
Absent 100	7 (38,9%)	93 (70,5%)
		p $<$0,001

This table shows a statistically significant correlation between the presence of DR 3 and proteinuria induced by gold salts.

CONCLUSIONS

This study has enable us to identify a high percentage of adverse reactions caused by therapy with these drugs.

Stomatitis and dermatitis were the adverse reactions more often observed and the reintroduction in a lower dosage in those patients who presented adverse reactions was sucessful in some cases.

There were no cases of adverse reactions leading to death.

The immunogenetic studies may open new vistas of the characterisation of patients who may develop adverse reactions with drugs.

It is probable that antigen DR 3 is related to proteinuria induced by gold salts, as B 27 is related to agranulocytosis induced by levamisol.

REFERENCES

Arrigoni-Martelli, E. (1982). Antirheumatic drugs. Drugs of Today, Vol. XVIII, no. 9, 461-508.

Batchelor, Jr. (1979). Genetics of Rheumatoid Arthritis. In Panayi G.S., Johnson P.M.: Imunopathogenesis of Rheumatoid Arthritis.

Crawhall, J.C. et al. (1963). Effects of penicillamine in cystinuria. Brit. Med. J. 1: 588.

Decker, J.C. (1977). The management of Rheumatoid Arthritis. Med. Times, 105: 28.

Deering, T.B. et al. (1977). Effect of D-penicillamine on copper retention in patients with primary biliary cirrhosis. Gastroenterology 72: 1208.

Dukes, M.N.G. (1981). Side effects of drugs. 9th Ed. Excerpta Medica.

E.R.C. Empire Rheumatium Council. (1961). Gold therapy in Rheumatoid Arthritis: Final report of a multicentre controled trial. Ann. Rheum. Dis. 20: 315-333.

Forrestier, J. (1934). Rheumatoid Arthritis and its treatment by gold salts. Lancet 2: 646-648.

Franchimont, P. et al. (1978). Adverse reactions to the principal drugs used in Rheumatoid Arthritis - A review. J. Rheumat. 5 (Suppl. 4): 85-92.

Fraser, T.N. (1945). Gold treatment in Rheumatoid Arthritis. Ann. Rheum. Dis. 4: 71.

Giroud, J.P., Mathé, G., Meyniel, G. (1978). Pharmacologie clinique. Bases de la thérapeutique. Paris. Ed. Expansion Scientifique Française.

Goodman, G.A., Goodman, L.S., Gilman, A. (1980). The pharmacological basis of therapeutics. 6th ed. New York. Ed.: Goodman and Gilman.

Hansten, P.D. Drug interactions. 4th ed. Philadelphia, Ed. Lea and Febiger.

Hill, Alan G.S. General management of Rheumatoid Arthritis in copeman's textbook of the rheumatic diseases. Ed. J.T. Scott (5th ed.).

Huskisson, E.C. (1978). The place of levamisol in the armamentarium for Rheumatoid Arthritis. J. Rheumat. 5 (Suppl. 4): 149-152.

Huskisson, E.C. et al. (1980). An overview of the current status of levamisol in the treatment of rheumatic diseases. Drugs 19:100-104.

Huskisson, E.C. (1981). Side effects of penicillamine therapy in RA. J. Rheumat. (Suppl. 7) 8: 146-148.

Jaffe, I.A. (1963). Comparison of the effect of plasma phoresis and peni-
    cillamine on the level of circulating rheumatoid factor.
    Ann. Rheum. Dis. 22: 71.

Jaffe, I.A. (1977-78). D-penicillamine. Bull. Rheum. Dis. 28: 948-952.

Katz et al. (1968). Comprehensive outpatient care in Rheumatoid Arthritis:
    a controled study. Jama 206: 1244.

Klinefelter, H.F. (1975). Reinstitution of gold therapy in Rheumatoid Ar-
    thritis after mucocutaneus reactions. J. Rheumat. 2: 21-27.

Kodda-Kimble, M.A., Katcher, B.S., Young, L.J. Applied therapeutics for
    clinical pharmacists. 2nd ed. San Francisco. Ed. Mary-Anne
    Kodda-Kimble.

Lawrence, J.S. (1970). Rheumatoid Arthritis. Annals of the Rheumatic
    Diseases, 29. 357-359.

Lightfoot, R.J. Treatment of Rheumatoid Arthritis. In Arthritis and Allied
    Conditions. Ed. Daniel J. McCarty (9th edition).

Mielants, H. et al. (1978). A study of hematological side effects of le-
    vamisol in Rheumatoid Arthritis. J. Rheumat. 5 (Suppl. 4):
    77-83.

Panayi et al. (1978). Genetic basis of rheumatoid disease: HLA antigens,
    disease manifestations and toxic reactions of drugs. Brit.
    Med. J., 1326-1328.

Rodnam, G.P. et al. (1970). The early story of rheumatic drugs. Arthritis
    Rheum. 13: 145.

Schattenkirscher, M. La chrysothérapie de la polyarthrite rhumatoide.
    Compendia Rheumatologica. Bâle. Ed. Eular.

Schwermans, Y. (1975). Levamisol in Rheumatoid Arthritis. Lancet I: 111.

Viana Queirós, M. et al. (1979). D-penicilamina no tratamento da Artrite
    Reumatóide. Jornal do Médico, CI, 1861: 383-385.

Wooley et al. (1980). HLA-DR antigens and toxic reactions to gold and
    d-penicillamine in patients with RA. N. Eng. J. Med., 303:
    300-303.

THE NUCLEAR MEDICINE TEAM

S Ellis.   Regional Pharmaceutical Officer
East Anglian Regional Health Authority, Cambridge, England

It is my pleasant duty to introduce the members of the nuclear medicine team from England who will outline their role in the planning and implementation of patient therapy.

Nuclear medicine is a relatively new specialty in hospital practice but it is growing rapidly both in the number of hospitals with a department and also in the breadth of its contribution to both diagnosis and treatment.

The radio-active nature of the pharmaceuticals used and the sophisticated equipment necessary for their application and measurement of results introduce several unique features into any nuclear medicine team.

Firstly the location in which they work. In order to protect staff and other patients in the hospital from exposure to radio-activity and because of the immobility of the monitoring equipment it is usual to confine the use of radio-pharmaceuticals to one area of the hospital and patients are taken to the team rather than the team visiting the wards.

Secondly extra safety precautions must be taken when handling radio-pharmaceuticals. Not only must the product be protected from micro-biological or cross contamination but those handling them must be protected from excess exposure to radioactivity. Thus the pharmacist will normally work within a clean environment provided with special safety cabinets, of the vertical laminar flow type, and situated in the nuclear medicine department away from the main pharmacy.

Thirdly it dictates the composition of the team because the scientific and technical problems which may be encountered require expertise outside that available on the usual health care team, namely that of physicists and technicians.

Today we are going to hear from three members of a team from the Department of Nuclear Medicine, Addenbrooke's Hospital, Cambridge.

Mr Barber, Senior Physicist and Dr Buxton-Thomas, Senior Registrar in that
department are joined by a former colleague Dr McCarthy who was Principal
Radiopharmacist on the team until she joined Travenol here in Belgium
last year.

They will describe the contribution they each make to the production and use of radio-pharmaceuticals for diagnostic and therapeutic
purposes.

PRACTICE OF THE NUCLEAR MEDICINE THERAPEUTIC TEAM

The Role of the Physicist

R. W. Barber
Department of Nuclear Medicine, Addenbrooke's Hospital, Hills
Road, Cambridge, CB2 2QQ

INTRODUCTION

Nuclear medicine may be defined as the application of
radioactive materials to the diagnosis and treatment of patients and the
study of human disease. The rapid growth of nuclear medicine into a
recognised medical discipline has required the close cooperation of
clinicians, physicists, technicians and pharmacists and the application of
a wide range of scientific and technical skills. Much of the importance
of nuclear medicine lies in the ability not only to aid the establishment
of a diagnosis, but also to assist in the therapeutic management of the
patient. The scope of nuclear medicine in   diagnosis and therapy is
summarised in table 1.

Table 1

THE SCOPE OF NUCLEAR MEDICINE
IN DIAGNOSIS AND TREATMENT

DIAGNOSIS:

IN VIVO	IN VITRO
Organ imaging	Measurement of pools and spaces
Organ function studies	biochemical analysis
Whole body imaging	assay of enzymes and hormones (Radioimmunoassay R.I.A.)
Whole body retention studies	
Blood flow measurements	

THERAPY

Malignant and non malignant disease

THE SCOPE OF NUCLEAR MEDICINE

Although nuclear medicine is primarily a diagnostic specialty, the initial events that spurred the growth of nuclear medicine technology were in therapeutic applications. Table 2 summarises how these complementary aspects of nuclear medicine combine to contribute to the overall management of the patient. Firstly, in establishing what is wrong with the patient, and the extent of the disease. Secondly, in outlining organs and delineating lesions. Such information for example can be used to guide treatment by external beam radiotherapy, or to aid biopsy. Thirdly, in treating the disease directly, possibly in combination with chemotherapy, external beam radiotherapy or surgery. Lastly, in evaluating the results of treatment and detecting recurrence of disease.

Table 2

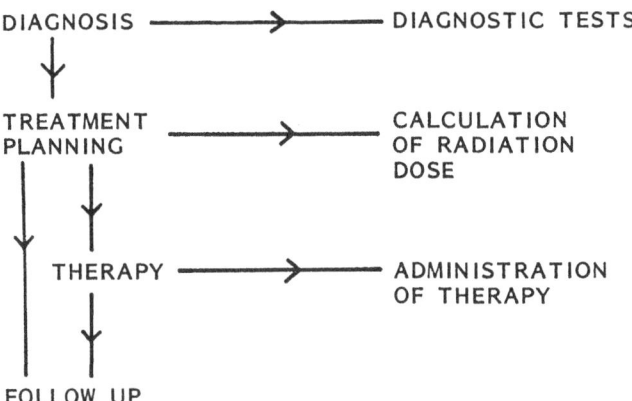

NUCLEAR MEDICINE IN PATIENT MANAGEMENT

DIAGNOSIS ⟶ DIAGNOSTIC TESTS

TREATMENT PLANNING ⟶ CALCULATION OF RADIATION DOSE

THERAPY ⟶ ADMINISTRATION OF THERAPY

FOLLOW UP

A few definitions are introduced in table 3 for those
unfamiliar with the terminology.

THE SPECIFICATION OF THE RADIOPHARMACEUTICAL

It is clearly important to specify the requirements of a
radiopharmaceutical both in terms of the physical characteristics of the
radionuclide used as the "label", and in terms of the pharmaceutical
itself. In diagnosis for example, the agent is not expected to elicit a
pharmacological effect. Indeed it is most important that it acts as a
true "tracer" and does not alter the physiology of the patient. The
radionuclide is chosen to be compatible with the imaging or other
instrumentation used while minimising the radiation dose to the patient.
When using a radiopharmaceutical in therapy, the therapeutic response is
due to a radiation effect, not a pharmacological one. It is necessary
to deliver a prescribed radiation dose to a given organ or tumour, while
sparing the adjacent normal tissue. The pharmacist needs to provide an
organ- or tumour-specific pharmaceutical: the physicist needs to provide
a radionuclide with the required physical characteristics.

Table 3

NUCLIDE   A version of a chemical element defined
               in terms of the structure of its nucleus

RADIONUCLIDE

               A nuclide with an unstable nucleus (radio-
               active) emitting alpha, beta or gamma radiation.

ISOTOPES   Nuclides with same atomic number

RADIOPHARMACEUTICAL

               A radioactive drug that can be administered
               to humans for diagnostic or therapeutic
               purposes

The main methods of production of radionuclides are listed in table 4. The commonest radionuclides are obtained from nuclear reactors, either by separation of the fission products of uranium, or by direct neutron bombardment of suitable targets. Cyclotron produced radionuclides are less readily available, and tend to be more expensive. However, they constitute an important group within the nuclear medicine field. Finally, a very important group of short-lived radionuclides is produced in the radiopharmacy by separation from a longer lived parent in generator systems. A wide range of radionuclides is now commercially available.

Table 4

PRODUCTION OF RADIONUCLIDES

Separation of fission products

Reactor production by neutron irradiation

Cyclotron production by charged particle irradiation

Secondary production – generator systems

Table 5 outlines the factors affecting the choice of radionuclide.

Table 5

CHARACTERISTICS OF RADIONUCLIDES

Radiations emitted

> **Alpha,beta,gamma X**

> **Energy**

> **Relative abundance**

Half life

DIAGNOSIS

We turn now to the important field of organ imaging and in-vivo organ function studies. The instrument shown in figure 1 is a rectilinear scanner, a moving detector device which measures the distribution of a radiopharmaceutical in an organ by scanning backwards and forwards across the patient. The radioactivity detected can be displayed line by line, and an image or "scintigram" formed. A more versatile instrument is the gamma camera, shown in figure 2. It consists of a large, stationary detector which can form an image of the whole organ at once. When the gamma camera is connected to a computer, it is possible to acquire and store sequential images. After data analysis, the passage of a radiopharmaceutical through an organ can be followed. Such "dynamic studies" have been developed in a wide range of situations. Thus the gamma camera is able to determine both anatomical structure and organ function simultaneously.

Figure 1

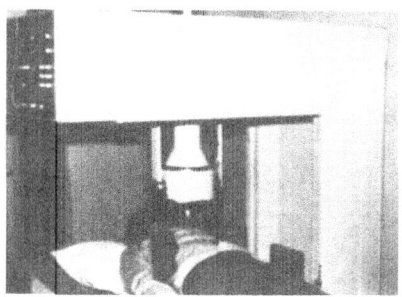

Figure 2

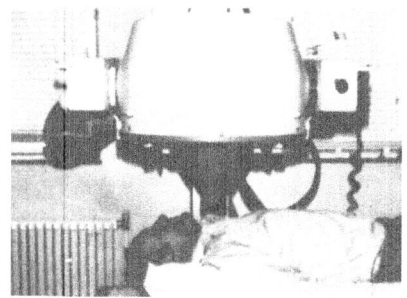

The requirements of a good diagnostic agent, suitable for organ imaging or in-vivo organ function studies are summarised in table 6. Firstly, the radionuclide should be primarily a gamma emitter: only gamma rays are penetrating enough to be visualised externally. Beta particles increase the tissue radiation dose without contributing useful information. Secondly, the energy of the gamma rays should be compatible with the radiation detector used. If the energy is too low, excessive amounts of absorption and scattering occur in the patient, and the image is degraded. If the energy is too high, the detector is insensitive. Thirdly, the physical half-life of the radionuclide should be long enough to allow accumulation of the agent in the organ of interest, and to allow measurements to be made, but not so long as to deliver an unacceptably high radiation dose. Lastly, the agent should be organ- or tumour-specific.

Table 6

REQUIREMENTS OF A GOOD IMAGING AGENT

Primary gamma emitting

Energy of gammas compatible with radiation detector (100 - 300 keV)

Short half life (few hours)

Organ/tumour specific

THERAPY

The main requirements of a therapeutic agent are listed in table 7. The radionuclide should be primarily a beta emitter.

Table 7

REQUIREMENTS OF A THERAPEUTIC AGENT

Primary Beta emitting (energetic betas)

Longish half-life   (few days)

Organ/tumour specific

The physical half-life of the radionuclide is usually of the order of a
few days. The contrast between the requirements for diagnosis and
therapy are clear. Of course, the radionuclide needs to be incorporated
into a suitable organ- or tumour-specific pharmaceutical.

The most convenient method to calculate radiation dose
following the administration of a radiopharmaceutical is the scheme
devised by the Medical Internal Radiation Dose (MIRD) Committee of the
U.S. Society of Nuclear Medicine. As can be seen in table 8, we are
required to estimate the energy deposited in unit mass of tissue. The
radiation dose depends on the biological behaviour of the pharmaceutical
and on the physical characteristics of the radionuclide. The MIRD scheme
provides a method of calculating the fraction of radiation energy
deposited in different organs under different situations for a wide range
of commonly used radionuclides. The MIRD scheme can be used to calculate
the amount of radioactivity that needs to be administered to deliver a
prescribed therapeutic radiation dose. It can also be used to estimate
the patient radiation dose from diagnostic procedures, and in assessing
the risks to staff handling radioactive materials.

Table 8

MEDICAL INTERNAL RADIATION DOSE (MIRD) CALCULATIONS

Biological data

    Distribution

    Uptake

    Clearance

    Mass of organ   m

Physical data

    Type of radiations

    Energy

    Half-life

    Absorbed fraction ϕ

$$D_t = \int_o^t A(t) \quad S\,(\phi, m)$$

Dose to time t   = cumulated activity x absorbed dose per
(energy absorbed   unit cumulated activity
per unit mass of
tissue)

The handling of all radioactive materials requires suitable precautions against contamination of staff or equipment, and a realisation that the patient is himself a source of external radiation. This is particularly important when dealing with the large activities of long lived materials used in therapy. In figure 3 we see a patient receiving a therapeutic dose of radioiodine: the clinical conditions under which this treatment is given will be described in the next paper. The radioiodine is contained within a rubber-capped vial inside a lead pot, and is despensed orally through a system of tubes. Staff wear rubber or plastic gloves to avoid contamination of the skin. Work is carried out over trays to contain the spread of contamination should a spill occur. Precautions are taken to avoid contaminating the patient's clothing. When larger amounts are given, it may be necessary to restrict the patient's movements with regard to travel by public transport or returning to work. When very large amounts are administered, as in carcinoma thyroid, it is necessary to admit the patient to hospital and segregate him in a side ward. The time spent with the patient by staff and visitors is kept to a minimum. The patient has his own toilet and washing facilities which are monitored on completion of his stay in hospital. He has his own crockery and cutlery which are also monitored before being allowed to be used by other patients. Decontamination is performed as necessary. The patient's bed linen may have to be washed separately.

It is also advisable to perform contamination checks on staff who handle radioactive materials, or who are in contact with patients who have received radiopharmaceuticals. Such checks are performed in a whole body monitor, shown in figure 4. This instrument consists of two very

Figure 3   Figure 4

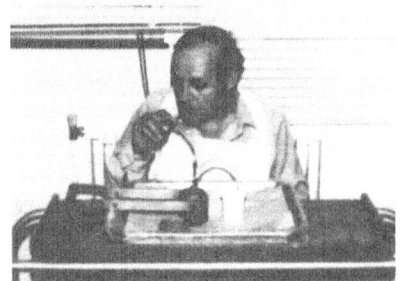

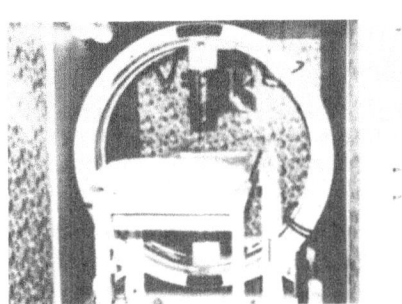

sensitive detectors contained within a shielded room to reduce the
natural background radiation. These checks are in addition to the usual
film badge monitoring.

CONCLUSION

In conclusion, the physicist plays a part in all aspects of
the handling of radioactive materials and the supervision of radiation
protection measures for patients and staff. His advice is sought on the
correct operation of the complex equipment used in nuclear medicine. He
is also involved in the design of diagnostic tests and the administration
of therapeutic amounts of radioactive materials.

PRACTICE OF THE NUCLEAR MEDICINE THERAPEUTIC TEAM

The Role of the Physician

M. S. Buxton-Thomas
Department of Nuclear Medicine, Addenbrooke's Hospital,
Hills Road, Cambridge, CB2 2QQ

INTRODUCTION

The physician in the therapeutic team is responsible for deciding on the best therapy for the patient and ensuring that this treatment is carried out. This would also involve monitoring the response to therapy and arranging for follow-up of the patient. This is achieved with the collaboration of clinician colleagues, physicists and technicians, and pharmacists: indeed, this teamwork forms the basis for the work of the department. This work involves primarily diagnostic imaging, but therapy forms a small, but nevertheless important, part. Occasionally, radiopharmaceuticals are used as therapy for certain haematological conditions, for example radioactive phosphorus in polycythaemia rubra vera. Also the intra-articular injection of colloids containing β emitting radionuclides has been used to control inflammation in joints. The radiation emitted locally causes destruction of the synovium resulting in a medical synovectomy. Currently ^{90}Yttrium, ^{186}Rhenium and ^{169}Erbium are the radionuclides in use. These emit β particles which are energetic to varying degrees and the radionuclide used in therapy depends on the thickness of the synovial membrane of the particular joint. However, it is in the management of thyroid disease that we play a large therapeutic role. This group of diseases will therefore serve as an illustration of the practice of the nuclear medicine therapeutic team.

DISEASES OF THE THYROID GLAND

They can be broadly divided into those due to

1. Overactivity of the gland - where excess hormone is produced and results in the clinical condition known as thyrotoxicosis or hyperthyroidism.

2. Underactivity of the gland - where not enough thyroid hormone is available for the body's needs and results in the clinical condition of myxoedema or hypothyroidism, and

3. Cancer or carcinoma of the gland.

There are other thyroid conditions but these three categories will serve for illustrative purposes.

THYROTOXICOSIS

In this condition, the patient might complain of weight loss, agitation, palpitations and swelling in the neck. The referring doctor requests a thyroid scan or scintigram so that information about the size and function of the gland can be obtained. Although the condition can be diagnosed from the results of biochemical tests, the appearances of the thyroid image obtained from the scan are often diagnostic.

Table 1

DISEASES OF THYROID GLAND

Due to:

1. Overactivity ⬆ T4 ⟶ Thyrotoxicosis or hyperthyroidism

2. Under-activity ⬇ T4 ⟶ Myxoedema or hypothyroidism

3. Carcinoma

4. Other e.g. infections,inflammatory and auto immune

For this investigation, the patient is given an intravenous injection of the radiopharmaceutical, usually 99mTc sodium pertechnetate, and images are made about 20 minutes later. The resulting image is shown on Figure 1.

In figure 1 both lobes of the gland are enlarged and there is uniformly high uptake of tracer or radiopharmaceutical. This is the typical appearance of Graves' disease, an example of thyrotoxicosis.

Figure 1

Graves' Disease

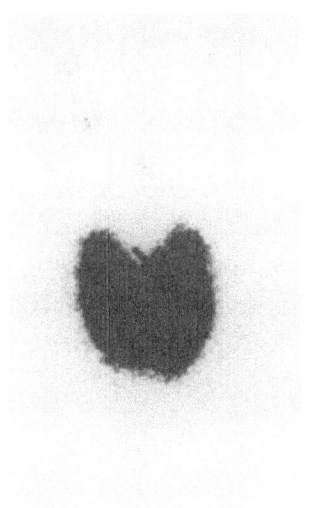

Another appearance that can be seen is shown in Figure 2. Here the patient has presented with the same symptoms previously described but the image obtained on the scan is different. There is high uptake in a palpable nodule. This nodule functions autonomously, that is without the control of the thyroid stimulating hormone (or TSH) produced from the pituitary gland and there is suppression of the remainder of the gland, the rest of the gland having little activity.

The image of the thyroid gland in another patient who again presented with similar symptoms of overactivity is shown in Figure 3. The appearances of the scintigram are again completely different. This time the gland is very large indeed with multiple regions of high activity suggestive of functioning nodularity. This gland is so large it extends below the neck and may, in certain situations, cause compression of the trachea. This information is important and has therapeutic implications as will be shown subsequently.

Figure 2   Figure 3

Autonomous 'Hot' Nodule   Multinodular Goitre with Retro-
                                                    sternal Extension

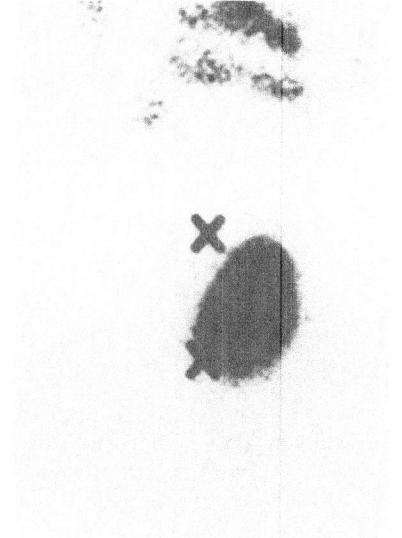

It can therefore be seen that, although these patients all
presented with the same symptoms of overactivity of the gland, the
scintigram appearances are different. It is essential to have the
information thus obtained from functional images, as therapy may be
different in the three situations. Our management of these conditions
will depend not only on the scintigraphic appearances, but also on other
clinical criteria. Some of the options available for the management of
thyrotoxicosis are summarised in Table 2. These include:-
1. Medical treatment - which involves the use of anti-thyroid drugs
and beta-blockers.
2. Surgical treatment - partial thyroidectomy.
One or other or both of these treatments can be offered to the younger
patient. However, there is a third method of treatment available which
is:
3. Radioiodine therapy.
This is generally reserved for the older patient. The treatment
strategy employed for the first example of thyrotoxicosis, that is
Graves' disease, would be medical treatment initially. If the patient
is young, then there may be a cure after some months. If this treatment
fails, then surgery can be offered.

In the middle-aged or older patient however, radioiodine
would be the suitable choice. In order to decide on the amount of
radioiodine to be administered, an attempt is made by the physicist to
assess the mass of the gland. This information, together with other
clinical and scintigraphic data, is used in determining the administered
activity.

Table 2

MANAGEMENT OF THYROTOXICOSIS

1. Medical - Antithyroid drugs and beta blockers

2. Surgical - Partial thyroidectomy

3. Radioiodine therapy

In the patient with the autonomous hyperfunctioning nodule, radioiodine therapy is recommended even if the patient is young. The amount of radioactivity administered here is usually larger than in the previous case.

In the third example, that of the very large gland compressing the trachea, one would take the precaution of admitting this patient. Medical treatment would be started initially and the antithyroid drugs are then stopped for a few days before radioiodine therapy is administered, to allow the blocking effects of these drugs to diminish. This allows sufficient uptake and trapping of the administered radioiodine.

In the initial period after therapy there may be temporary swelling of the gland which could cause partial or complete obstruction of the trachea. Having the patient in hospital ensures that medical staff are on hand to deal with this situation should it arise.

Surgical decompression by removal of part of the gland is another alternative.

In the second group of thyroid diseases, that is in underactivity of the gland, the department is not usually involved on the therapeutic side. This is because treatment simply involves replacing the patient's hormone requirements with thyroxine tablets and any other symptomatic treatment that is required.

THYROID CARCINOMA

However, in the third group of diseases - carcinoma of the thyroid - nuclear medicine is involved in all three aspects of diagnosis, therapy and follow-up. Here, the possibility of carcinoma is often raised by the scintigraphic appearance. The patient may notice a hard swelling in the neck, and the scintigram could have the appearance shown in Figure 4.

Figure 4
'Cold' Nodule

In this case there is no uptake of tracer (and therefore no functioning thyroid tissue) in part of the right lobe, where the swelling is situated. This is usually referred to as a 'cold' nodule. Further investigation needs to be carried out as although the appearance is suspicious of a carcinoma, it is not diagnostic, and other conditions such as a cyst would give similar appearances. However, if the diagnosis of carcinoma is established, usually after a biopsy, surgical treatment is recommended. At operation, the surgeon would attempt to remove the tumour and as much of the gland as possible.

Post-operatively, we would become involved in the further assessment of the patient, if histological examination reveals that there are functioning thyroid cells in the tumour. Follow-up whole body scintigrams using ^{131}I-Iodide as the radiopharmaceutical, are then performed at intervals. This radiopharmaceutical is used, as it is specific for functioning thyroid tissue, and will give information about the growth and spread of the tumour, and is itself the therapeutic agent when used in larger amounts. An example of a patient with thyroid carcinoma is shown in Figure 5. A total thyroidectomy had been performed and the six month follow-up ^{131}Iodine scintigram shows multiple regions of high uptake particularly in the lungs.

Figure 5
^{131}I Scintigram
Carcinoma of Thyroid with Metastases

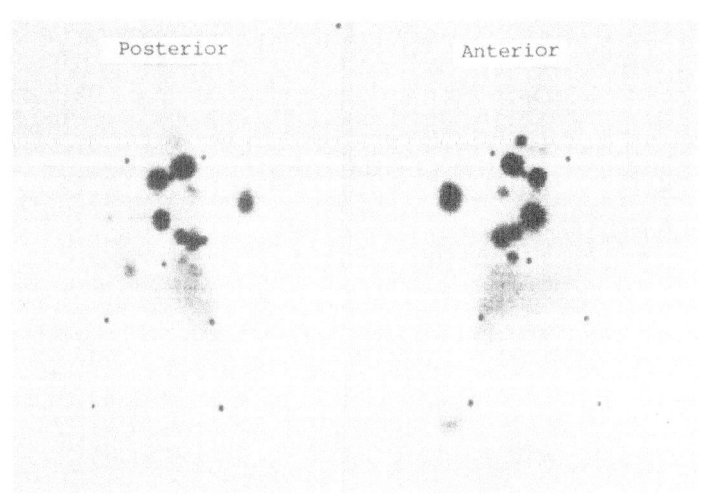

In Figure 6 the same patient's chest x-ray for comparison does not show up the secondary tumours in the lungs very well. Having confirmed that there is spread of the tumour, the patient can be given a second radioiodine drink - this time, therapeutic, and usually a very large amount. After a few months, the ^{131}Iodine whole body scintigram can be repeated to assess the response to therapy.

Figure 6

^{131}I Scintigram   Chest X-ray

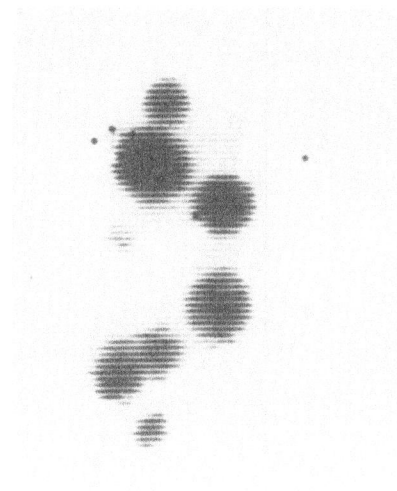 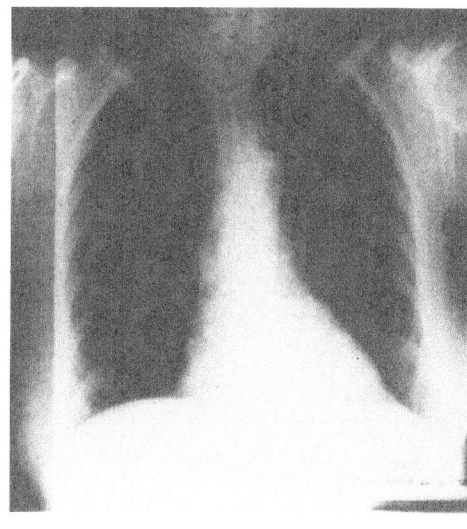

CONCLUSION

These are the main clinical situations in which nuclear medicine is directly involved with therapy. As mentioned by the previous speaker, the large part of our work is in diagnostic functional imaging but these will then have therapeutic consequences. The physician ensures that the patient is cared for while in the department and that the necessary diagnostic information is obtained, and where necessary, the best therapy instituted. This therapeutic effect however is not pharmacological, but produced by a radiation effect.

The future for radiopharmacy is exciting as not only are organ specific agents being produced but also cell-specific ones.

It is now possible to label antibodies to certain tumour types with the aim of not only imaging them for diagnostic purposes but also with a view to therapy. A new radiopharmaceutical is now available for imaging adrenal medullary tumours which can also be used in therapy.

PRACTICE OF THE NUCLEAR MEDICINE THERAPEUTIC TEAM

The Role of the Radiopharmacist

T. McCarthy, previously Addenbrooke's Hospital, now Travenol, Belgium

In illustrating the role of the radiopharmacist in the
Nuclear Medicine team - where better to start than with the radiopharmaceuticals. To re-emphasise what has been said already:

A radiopharmaceutical is a substance intended for human
administration which has been modified by the incorporation
of a radionuclide. Dependant on the type of radiation
emitted and the chemical form, the radiopharmaceutical may
be suitable for a variety of therapeutic or diagnostic uses.

Unlike most other drugs, radiopharmaceuticals are administered
in very small (often nanogram) amounts and are not desired to have any
pharmacological effect. The chemical or pharmaceutical moiety should
however, be organ or function specific so that the radionuclide which it
carries, can be used for selective imaging or target specific radiotherapy.

Although Nuclear Medicine is a discipline encompassing both
diagnostic and therapeutic roles the major role to date, other than in
the treatment of some thyroid, haematological and a few rheumatological
disorders, has been in the use of radiopharmaceuticals to facilitate
diagnosis and to monitor therapy. Nuclear Medicine aids not only in the
selection of the correct therapy be it surgery or drugs, but also
provides a means of avoiding some potentially unpleasant therapy where
treatment is inappropriate. An ideal example is the use of radiopharmaceuticals in determining the presence of secondary metastases in
e.g. bone or liver before deciding on the treatment of a primary lung
carcinoma. (X-ray techniques are of course also complimentary here in
detecting secondary spread). Since Nuclear Medicine tests are themselves
atraumatic, involving little more than an intravenous injection, a
waiting period, and the need to lie still during imaging - the benefits
are enormous.

To understand fully the radiopharmacist's role one must however know something more about radiopharmaceuticals. As this symposium is for pharmacists from different pharmaceutical disciplines - I will initially review some of the basics of radiopharmacy. Although we are now seeing increasing use of more radionuclides such as Indium-111, Iodine-123 and Gallium-67, the most commonly used nuclides in Nuclear Medicine today are still, Technetium 99m and Iodine-131 (Table 1).

The material with which everyone outside Nuclear Medicine will be most familiar is of course iodine which has an obvious use in the management of thyroid disorders, being selectively concentrated in this gland. Since iodine-131 decays with the emission of both beta and gamma rays it can be used in both therapy and diagnosis. For diagnostic studies however, the energy of the gamma rays is not ideal for the detectors and the presence of beta particles results in unnecessary radiation dose to the patient. Generator produced technetium 99m a pure gamma emitter of short half life is therefore a preferred nuclide for diagnostic studies.

Table 1

NUCLIDE	CHARACTERISTIC RADIATION	ENERGY (keV)	HALF LIFE	SOURCE
TECHNETIUM-99m	gamma	140	6 hours	GENERATOR
IODINE - 131	gamma - - - - - -	364	8 days	REACTOR
	beta - - - - - -	.606		

A supply of technetium 99m can be obtained from a radionuclide generator, Figure 1. The generator is a system for separating the short-lived Technetium 99m from its longer-lived parent, Molybdenum 99. The parent is radioactive and will decay to produce a continuous supply of the daughter nuclide which can be eluted at appropriate intervals. Figure 2 shows the build-up of technetium from decay of Molybdenum followed by elution and regrowth.

<u>Figure 1</u>

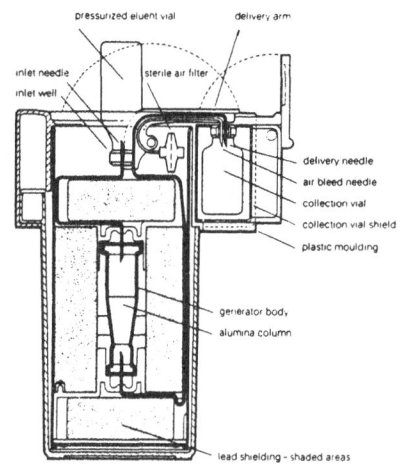

<u>Figure 2</u>

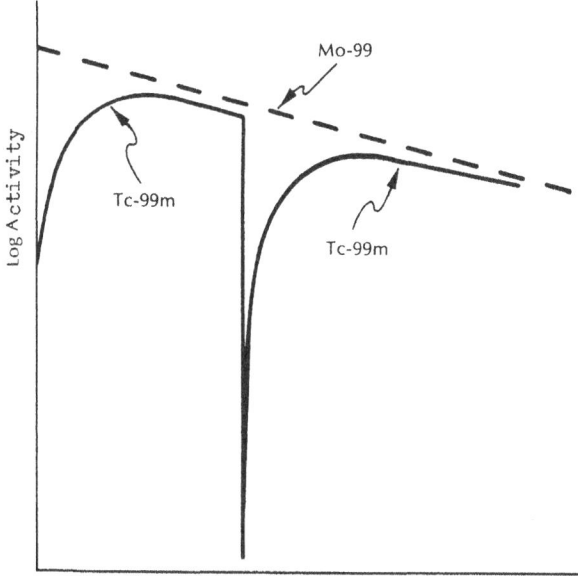

Technetium 99m is eluted from a generator in the seven
oxidation state as a solution of sodium pertechnetate in sodium chloride.
Since it has approximately the same ionic volume as iodide the
pertechnetate ion will be concentrated in the thyroid, and salivary
glands, secreted in the gastric mucosa, and excluded from the brain by
the blood brain barrier. It can be used in both thyroid and brain
imaging. The thyroid is visualised as an area of increased radioactivity
against a cold background in figure 3, whereas the brain, figure 4, is
seen as a region of low activity in which abnormalities appear hot. For
most other investigations Technetium 99m must be linked (generally
following reduction) to a variety of other pharmaceutical agents in
order to achieve selective localisation in the organ of interest.

Figure 3   Figure 4

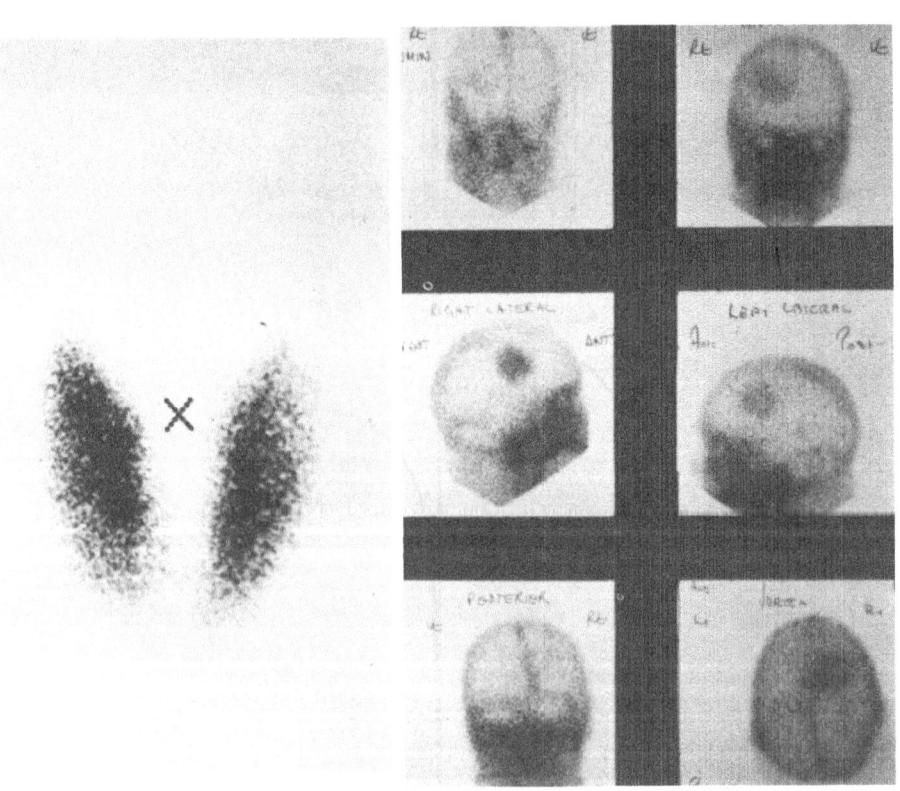

Some of the agents to which Technetium 99m is linked for
various investigations are listed below:

Albumin microspheres	for Lung Perfusion imaging
Sulphur colloid	for Liver imaging
Antimony sulphide colloid	for Internal Mammary lymph node imaging
Methylene diphosphonate	for Skeletal imaging
Diethylene triamine penta acetic acid	for Kidney studies
Iminodiacetic acid	for Hepatobiliary imaging
and Red Cells	for Blood pool studies of the heart

An obvious role for the radiopharmacist is therefore the
supply of these materials in a safe and effective form.

The quality of a radiopharmaceutical can significantly affect
its value in diagnosis. In addition to the parameters controlled for
non-radioactive drugs it is also necessary to control both radionuclidic
and radiochemical purity. The Radionuclidic Purity is the fraction of
the total activity present in the form of the desired radionuclide. The
Radiochemical Purity is the fraction of the total activity present in the
required chemical form.

Radionuclidic purity, must be controlled predominantly for
radiation safety reasons. Since technetium 99m is obtained from a
generator the most likely radionuclidic impurity in sodium pertechnetate
for instance would be the parent nuclide Molybdenum 99. As Molybdenum 99
decays with the emission of beta particles and has a 67 hour half life
the presence of even a small amount of Molybdenum in the Technetium 99m
could significantly increase the radiation dose to the patient. Table 2
shows the vast difference in radiation dose to the liver from equal
activities of both of these nuclides when Tc99m sulphur colloid is contaminated with Molybdenum.

Table 2

Comparative Radiation Dose to the Liver from Parent and Daughter Nuclides given Intravenously	
Molybdenum 99 (molybdate)	14 mSv MBq^{-1}
Technetium 99m (sulphur colloid)	$0.08 \text{ mSv MBq}^{-1}$

Whilst radionuclidic purity is primarily important from the radiation dosimetry standpoint, radiochemical purity is also important for the accurate interpretation of a scan. The very basis of the use of radiopharmaceuticals is their selective localisation in the organ of interest. The presence of other labelled molecules with different localisation characteristics would make the interpretation of activity distribution highly complex. Since the starting material for all Technetium 99m labelled radiopharmaceuticals is sodium pertechnetate the most likely impurity in for instance Technetium labelled methylene diphosphonate, albumin microspheres or sulphur colloid would be free pertechnetate. Figure 5 and 6 show visualisation of the thyroid on a lung scan due to the presence of free pertechnetate and visualisation of the stomach on a bone scan. Such extreme examples are rarely seen but can occur if care is not taken.

Figure 5   Figure 6

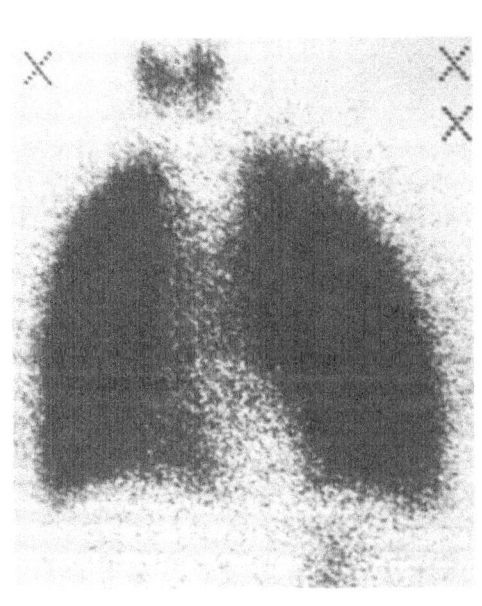
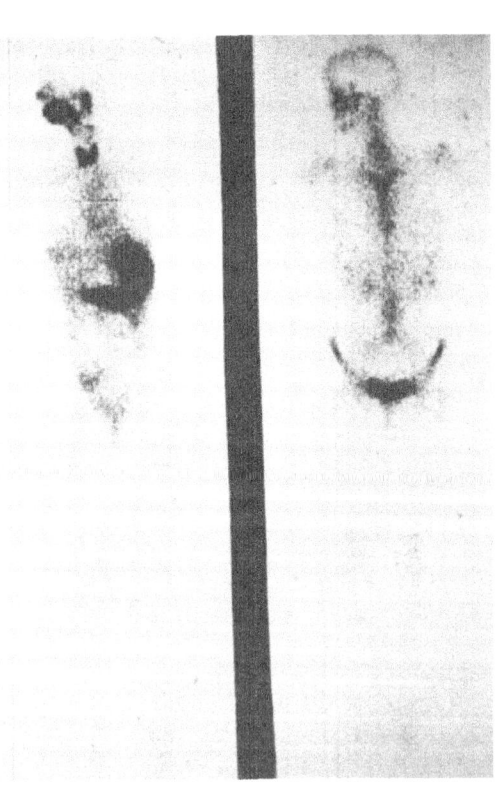

Many of the radiopharmaceuticals referred to above are now prepared from kit reagents and despite the complex chemistry involved, their preparation involves little more than aseptic transference and minor manipulative procedures. The quality is fairly easy to control and the hazards of handling them minimised by the use of well designed facilities and good techniques and procedures.

Apart from the routine preparation of established material from kits one very important role of the radiopharmacist in the Nuclear Medicine team in the research and development of new, improved radio-pharmaceuticals. This research often takes place in the hospital laboratory and a more complex procedure is involved.

Over the past few years there has been a significant increase in the number of procedures in which a patient's own cells are radio-labelled and used in imaging studies. The problems in labelling red cells with Technetium 99m are now fairly well resolved and great improvements have been made in labelling white cells with Indium-111.

This particular preparation was a very interesting one since problems were experienced in achieving efficient labelling without loss of viability of the cells. Separation of the white cells from whole blood was necessary because the labelling technique was not specific for those cells and yet this very separation significantly decreased the viability of the white cells and changed their distribution. Radio-labelled Indium was originally supplied as a chloride and had to be linked to oxine itself and heavy metal impurities such as cadmium which can be present in the Indium are toxic and these decreased cell viability still further. Finally when efficient labelling was achieved the benefits of high specific activity labelling of the cells had to be balanced against the radiation damage to the cells. Many of these problems are now resolved and a kit preparation is available so that the procedure is easier and the quality of the product is of a reproducible high standard. In this particular case the use of a nuclide other than Technetium was needed to produce the required radiopharmaceutical.

Although pharmacists are still attempting to label some compounds with Technetium 99m this nuclide has significant limitation for labelling biologically active molecules and attention is again turning to isotopes of iodine in an attempt to improve specificity. Iodine 123 amphetamine is now being explored for brain imaging and

Iodine 131 labelled meta iodobenzyl guanidine (MIBG) being developed for
pheochromocytoma. This analogue of guanethidine, Figure 7, is taken
up into adrenergic vesicles due to its similarity in structure to
Noradrenaline and facilitates diagnosis and localisation of
pheochromocytoma which is a potentially life threatening disorder.

At present the manipulations required to prepare MIBG are
quite complex. However, it can be made labelled with Iodine 123 or
Iodine 131 and therefore has potential use in both diagnosis and therapy
if the required purity is achieved and selectivity assured.

Certain tumour specific monoclonal antibodies have now been
produced and attempts are being made to label these with Iodine 131,
initially for diagnosis but potentially also for therapy. Thus we have
come full circle. Nuclear Medicine started with the use of Iodine 131
in therapy extended to the use of this and other nuclides in diagnosis
and now sees the possibility of tumour specific agents labelled with
Iodine 131 for both diagnosis and therapy. All that is required is a
safe and appropriate radiopharmaceutical. The radiopharmacist's role is
therefore clear.

Figure 7

ADRENOMEDULLARY AGENT

I - 131 META-IODOBENZYL GUANIDINE (MIBG)

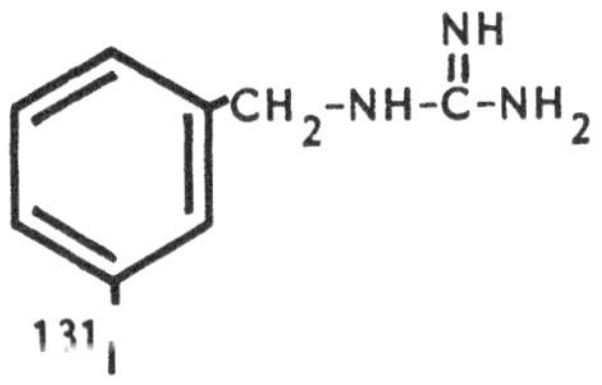

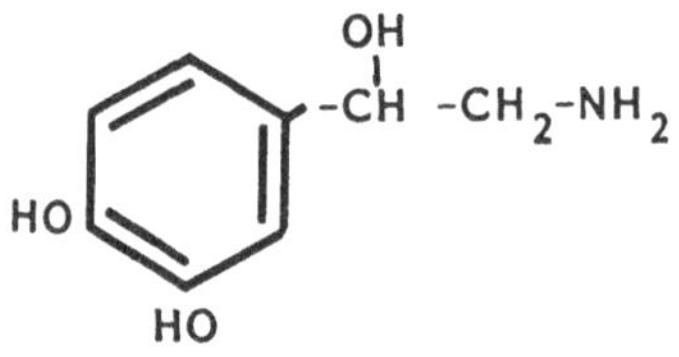

$$\text{CH}_2-\text{NH}-\overset{\overset{\displaystyle \text{NH}}{\|}}{\text{C}}-\text{NH}_2$$

^{131}I

$$-\overset{\overset{\displaystyle \text{OH}}{|}}{\text{CH}} -\text{CH}_2-\text{NH}_2 \quad \text{NORADRENALINE}$$

(for comparison)

HO

HO

COLLABORATION IN DRUG SELECTION - PREPARING THE LONDON HOSPITAL
FORMULARY 1982 - GUIDE TO THE PRESCRIBING OF MEDICINES

C.W. Barrett, et al.
The Pharmacy Department, The London Hospital (Whitechapel),
London, E1 1BB, England

INTRODUCTION

C.W. Barrett

Formularies were commonplace among the larger hospitals in
Great Britain in the latter half of the nineteenth century and the early
part of the twentieth century. They provided prescribers with a range of
formulations and rules for prescribing. The main reason for their exist-
ence was to control the large amount of preparative work required by the
Pharmacy and a secondary reason was to control expenditure.

These Formularies went out of use during the Second World War
and were largely replaced in post-war years by the British National
Formulary (BNF). As the therapeutic explosion of the 1950s and 60s
gained momentum the BNF, which was revised every four to five years,
gradually lost credibility because it did not keep pace with therapeutic
advances. This was corrected in 1981 by the publication of a new style
BNF, revised editions of which are now being produced at intervals of six
months.

In the 1960s in America the preparation of local formularies
gained momentum and this trend developed, albeit more slowly, in some
European countries during the 1970s. The recent trend to produce local
formularies in Britain has been paralleled by the increasing activities
of hospital drug and therapeutic committees and the increasing pressures
on resources.

WHY LOCAL FORMULARIES?

Given that local formularies are time consuming and expensive
to prepare and update and given that the BNF has now been considerably
improved the question must be asked why local formularies? The main
reason is simply that the range of drugs used in most hospitals is unacceptably large. A secondary reason is that they can be seen as a
constructive influence on containing drug expenditure. The range of drugs
in most hospitals varies between two and a half and three and a half
thousand and there is, therefore, a very significant proliferation of

preparations with basically similar clinical applications. It is becoming increasingly difficult for doctors, pharmacists and nurses to work safely, knowledgably and efficiently within this large range and at a time of severe financial constraint it does not make sense to perpetuate this situation with its consequent unnecessary cost implications. Local formularies are, therefore, considered necessary to reduce this range to an acceptable level, to provide necessary supportive information on the drugs included, to provide information on local drug use policies and guidance and to contain cost.

HOW PREPARATION OF THE FORMULARY WAS APPROACHED

Although in Great Britain clinicians still have complete freedom to prescribe whatever drug they consider most suitable for their patient, there is a growing recognition of the need for guidance. Pharmacists have a peculiar double responsibility. The paramount one is a professional responsibility to ensure as far as they reasonably can that the drugs they supply are safe and will be used safely and effectively. The second responsibility which cannot override the first responsibility is to purchase and supply drugs as cost effectively as possible within the constraints and limitations of the organisation.

In preparing The London Hospital Formulary 1982 - Guide To The Prescribing Of Medicines the three requirements in the paragraph above have had to be very carefully taken into account so that they are kept in their proper perspective, so that neither group feels threatened, and so that available resources are used to maximum benefit. The preparation of individual chapters was undertaken by teams of expert doctors and pharmacists who had the additional responsibility of confirming that the drafts produced were acceptable to their colleagues. How doctors and pharmacists approached this task will now be described.

A CLINICIAN'S VIEW ON THE TEAM APPROACH TO DRUG SELECTION

C.R. Darley
Department of Dermatology, The London Hospital (Whitechapel),
London E1 1BB, England

I would like to discuss some of the factors which influenced drug selection in the dermatological section of our formulary. The principal aim was to produce clear and simple guidelines for non-specialists. Firstly the drug must be effective and established, two points which may not by synonymous. New drugs need to be fully appraised before they are included, while a critical look at established preparations should be made in case newer products are more appropriate. Ketoconazole and Griseofulvin, both drugs used in the systemic treatment of ringworm infections provide us with an example. At the moment there is no evidence that Ketoconazole is significantly more effective than Griseofulvin in the treatment of this kind of infection. Griseofulvin is certainly well established while Ketoconazole is not. Ketoconazole was, therefore, not included in the present formulary but the relationship between these two drugs must be reviewed for future editions.

The spectrum of action of topical preparations is particularly important in relation to antimicrobial agents. For example, the imidazole compounds are effective against dermatophytes, yeasts and certain bacteria. This simplifies the choice although the established position of nystatin in the treatment of pure candida infections remains unchanged.

Resistance of organisms to topical and systemic antibacterial and antifungal agents must be taken into account. There may be antibacterial resistance policies to be considered. In the formulary under discussion topical antibiotics which are potentially useful systemically, such as Fusidic acid and Gentamicin are not included.

Potency is particularly important when considering topical corticosteroids. These are now graded into four groups according to potency, so any selection should include a preparation from each group.

The adverse effects of the drugs chosen should be infrequent and mild. In dermatological therapeutics the range of adverse effects are

small but they are all too evident to the patient when they do occur.
Popular topical preparations seldom cause significant irritation. What
is more important is the frequency with which a chemical applied to the
skin is likely to induce sensitisation and a contact dermatitis. Topical
antihistamines, local anaesthetics and some antibiotics are not used by
dermatologists because they are such common sensitisers. Neomycin is a
less common sensitiser, but the frequency with which it causes problems
is such that it was not included in the formulary under discussion.

     Although warning about contraindications can be included in
the text, it is desirable to choose preparations which have few such
problems. Drugs which might harm the patient by injudicious use or by
application in the wrong disease or site should be avoided as far as
possible.

     The amount of time spent by dermatological patients in the
application of their treatment is considerable. Non-compliance is
probably much more common than we admit so every effort should be made to
simplify treatment. This is not always possible as, for example, in the
treatment of scabies. Cosmetically unacceptable preparations will also
result in non-compliance. Very messy preparations such as Dithranol in
Lassar's paste are seldom a practical treatment for outpatients. Some of
the coloured substances which stain may also be avoided.

     Economic considerations are secondary to effective and safe
treatment but important savings may be made. As far as possible the
least expensive of comparable alternatives should be chosen. Dilutions
and non-standard mixtures should generally be avoided. They offer few
advantages to the specialist, they tend to confuse non-specialists and
they occupy considerable pharmacy time. Educational points in the
formulary may have beneficial economic consequences. Careful prescribing
and patient instructions reduce wastage. Family doctors and hospital non-
specialists may be encouraged to follow therapeutic advice in the
formulary. This may save hospital specialist time in the long term.

     The safety and educational aspects of the formulary are
inseparable. It is directed towards the non-specialist and simplicity
and clarity should be the aim. If this is fulfilled, the formulary may
also be valuable to student nurses and doctors.

     Indications for the use of different drugs should be clearly
delineated whether they be wide or narrow. Thus, on the one hand, topical
Salicylic acid may be used in a number of hyperkeratotic conditions while,

on the other, Podophyllin paint should only be used on viral warts aris-
ing on mucous membranes.

The formulary provides an opportunity to remind doctors of the
spectrum of action of antimicrobial agents, a subject which we have
already mentioned. The varying potency of topical corticosteroids has
also been discussed briefly. This group of drugs are highly effective
and very widely used. As a result of the experience gained it is now
possible to suggest a list of precautions which allow their efficacy to
be fulfilled within an acceptable safety margin. Thus, particular
recommendations are made to restrict the use of the more potent preparations on the face, flexures and in children, while it is advised that the
most potent are avoided except for short periods.

Deciding on a topical or systemic preparation is a clinical
judgement which depends on a number of things including the severity of
the condition and the depth of skin involved in the disease process.

Important adverse effects must be enumerated. They may be
divided into immediate such as the irritant reaction which may be seen
after Podophyllin treatment, immediate and long term such as a contact
dermatitis due to Neomycin which remains with the patient throughout
their life and long term such as the changes which result from prolonged
use of potent topical corticosteroids on the face. Topical preparations
may be absorbed into the circulation and have identical adverse effects
to those seen after systemic administration.

Lists of contraindications of topical therapy must assume some
diagnostic skill on the part of the clinician to avoid becoming exhaustive.
However, important contraindications such as the avoidance of topical
corticosteroids in purely infective conditions should be included in the
text.

There are three types of heading used in the formulary under
discussion. This is necessary for completeness although some overlap is
inevitable. They are firstly, drug group (eg. topical corticosteroids),
secondly, drug action (eg. emollients), and thirdly, disease (eg. acne
vulgaris). Under the last of these headings the formulary loses its
format, but it is useful to cover the management of some of the common
skin diseases such as eczema and psoriasis. Readers may then refer back
to recommended drug groups for more detailed information.

Clarity and accuracy in dermatological prescribing is particularly important. The choice of vehicle or base will depend on the skin

site and the disease to be treated. The frequency of application should
be stated and in some cases the duration of application indicated. The
quantity to be supplied will depend on the area of skin involved. The
area to which the topical preparation is to be applied must be stated and
whether normal skin should be treated as well as abnormal skin. Special
instructions such as advice on bathing and warnings about staining and
other unpleasant properties should not be omitted.

Each section in the formulary is written by an expert in the
particular field. As such the compiler has the authority to consider
certain areas of therapeutics too specialised for the generalist. For
example the use of certain drugs may be discouraged by their omission
from the formulary. Systemic cytotoxic drugs in the treatment of
psoriasis were not included. It may be considered prudent to prohibit
other drugs. In the formulary under discussion it was stated that
systemic corticosteroids should not be used in skin diseases without
prior consultation with a dermatologist.

The formulary must be updated on a regular basis. New drugs
can be incorporated if they have definite advantages over older preparations. New indications or side effects of drugs already recommended may
become apparent. Medical and pharmacy staff should be encouraged to make
criticisms and suggestions. Above all, the users of the formulary should
feel that changes can be made if there are good reasons.

Since the introduction of our formulary we have become aware
of an encouraging response on the part of clinicians and pharmacists.
It undoubtedly provides a safe and educational guide to the non-
specialist, while for the specialist, although no such limitations should
apply, the formulary provides a convenient and sound basis for treatment.

A PHARMACIST'S VIEW ON THE TEAM APPROACH TO DRUG SELECTION

A.C. Tugwell
Drug Information Centre, The London Hospital (Whitechapel),
London E1 1BB, England

This paper briefly outlines my views and experience as a
hospital pharmacist on the process of drug selection, in particular with
respect to the selection of drugs for a local formulary.

PRESCRIBING SITUATIONS

From the start, a distinction must be drawn between the various
prescribing situations that exist. These can broadly be divided into
three.

Firstly, the use of 'specialised' drugs by appropriate specialists which are not normally used by other clinicians; for example the use
of cytotoxic drugs by oncologists, or the use of general anaesthetic
agents.

Secondly, the situation where specialists are using drugs which
are also used by the non-specialist. A good example of this is the use of
dermatological preparations.

Lastly, the situation where a clinician wishes to treat disorders of a general nature when it is considered that specialist consultation may not be necessary.

This paper relates only to the last of these three situations.
Without some form of guidelines, this results in a large range of drugs
being used with all the problems that this entails which have been
previously outlined. At The London Hospital we have attempted to reduce
these problems with the introduction of a guide to the prescribing of
medicines which serves the purpose of a local formulary.

HOW DO PRESCRIBERS SELECT DRUGS?

How does a clinician in the last of the three situations that
I have just outlined decide which drug to prescribe? In many instances
he has a large number of possibilities. A quick examination of the
hypnotic drugs available in the United Kingdom shows that there are no
less than 20 to choose from; and there are currently 57 products for

hypertension available (22 of which contain a beta-blocker). So how does
he choose?

In the first instance, a prescriber chooses a drug after considering one
or more of the following:-

1. What he was taught while at medical college, although this is
   probably not a major factor.
2. Knowledge he has gained during his postgraduate training posts.
3. His preferences gained from his own clinical experience.
4. Local medical policies (if they exist).

Sometimes outside influences operate:-

1. What he has read in recent publications. This might tempt him
   into trying a drug which he would not otherwise have
   considered using.
2. What he has heard from colleagues or from attendance at
   clinical meetings.
3. Pressure from drug companies, either in the form of adverti-
   sing material or by the product-promoting activities of
   medical representatives.

Sometimes he seeks guidance:-

1. By asking a medical colleague.
2. By asking a pharmacist or a Drug Information Centre.
3. By referring to a reference book or other literature.
   HOW DO PHARMACISTS SELECT DRUGS?

A pharmacist chooses a drug after considering one or more of the
following:-

1. What he was taught at pharmacy college.
2. Impressions gained from medical colleagues.
3. Local drug policies (if they exist).
4. Other sources, for example, published information and data.
   Apart from the various manual retrieval systems available,
   many of the Drug Information Centres in Britain now have on-
   line computing facilities which enable pharmacists to examine
   the literature more thoroughly using the various files
   available, such as Medline and Excerpta Medica. Pharmacists
   in these centres with computerised retrieval systems are now
   in an even better position to carry out comprehensive studies
   into the various aspects which need to be considered, by
   reference to clinical trial data, toxicological data, and

comparative studies between different drugs. 'Other sources' also includes advice from clinicians or pharmacists who have particular knowledge in the area concerned.

Sometimes outside influences operate:-

1. Again, pressure from drug company representatives who obviously try to influence drug use within the hospital.

2. Pressure from the health authorities, who are always trying to save money, and to whom the chief pharmacist is directly accountable.

DRUG SELECTION CRITERIA FOR A FORMULARY

When making rational decisions on which drugs should be included in a formulary, certain criteria must be used in the selection process. It may well be the case, that one profession places more importance on some of the criteria than the other, however, both clinicians and pharmacists are primarily concerned with:-

EFFICACY - if a drug does not work there is little point in using it and no point in considering the other criteria.

SAFETY - this includes various aspects such as toxicity, side effects and potential safety problems related to contraindications, special precautions or interactions.

COST - this is of increasing importance in the United Kingdom, and is an aspect which hospital pharmacists in particular are concerned with since the chief pharmacist is the drug-budget holder and has responsibilities for promoting economical drug therapy. However, like clinicians it is important that pharmacists do not allow the first two criteria (ie. efficacy and safety) to become compromised on grounds of saving some money.

Although these are the prime cirteria which must be applied, there are other factors which must also be considered and these include:-

1. Ready availability of the drug both to hospitals and the community pharmacists.

2. Convenient and uncomplicated dosage regimes. If complicated, this can lead to poor patient compliance after their discharge from hospital.

3. Patient acceptability,

eg. size of tablets (and perhaps the number that need to be swallowed at each dose) taste

side effects

cosmetic (dermatological preparations)

4. Suitable range of routes of administration if appropriate.

5. Product stability.

eg. storage conditions required ⎫
    shelf-life   ⎬ eg. dermatology
    compatibility   ⎭

CLINICIAN/PHARMACIST COLLABORATION

Both professions are concerned with these factors, although as I have already indicated, some factors may be of more concern to one profession than the other.

There is also another difference. The approach in implementing these criteria often differs between the two professions. The clinician obviously puts a lot of weight on his views gained from personal experience in the success or otherwise of using certain drugs, whereas the pharmacist puts much emphasis on published data which stands up to critical evaluation and scrutiny.

So both professions want to achieve the same result, that is to select the best drugs for treatment by considering criteria such as efficacy and safety etc., but have different approaches in applying such criteria. This could lead to conflict - but it need not! In fact, it can often be quite healthy to have more than one approach to the same problem, providing everyone has the same objective. It is possible to prevent the situation where you have two interested parties becoming one of conflict, and instead adopting a team approach where each recognises and values the contribution of the other. We have shown that this can work well, and believe that balanced decisions are made by the clinician/pharmacist team which are also more readily accepted by practitioners of the professions concerned who will be affected.

So reviewing the advantages of this team approach in making drug selection decisions:-

1. All factors affecting choice are considered. It is unlikely that either profession individually would do so.

2. Balanced decisions are made, based both on published information and clinical experience (ie. objective and subjective contribution).

3. Acceptance of the decisions and policies made is much more

likely by practitioners of both professions.

SUPPORTING INFORMATION AND PRESENTATION

Lastly, I would like to emphasise the importance of providing
supportive information in the book to help in the effective and safe use
those drugs which have been selected for inclusion. In our 'Guide To The
Prescribing of Medicines' we give brief details on dosage, contraindications, interactions and side effects. We also have a 'comments'
section where any additional advice is given to ensure that the drugs
are used in the best possible way. This supporting information is
welcomed by users of the book and encourages them to prescribe the drugs
recommended. Like the drug selection process itself, it is equally
important that a team approach is adopted in preparing this information
for each section to ensure that it is technically correct and clinically
relevant.

The layout and design of a formulary must be considered to be
a crucial factor in deciding whether it will be used or not. The
information must be given in a clear and logical manner. Efforts made in
ensuring this are repaid in a willingness by the clinicians and
pharmacists to refer to the book since it is straightforward and easy to
use.

COLLABORATION IN DRUG SELECTION - PREPARING THE LONDON HOSPITAL
FORMULARY 1982 - GUIDE TO THE PRESCRIBING OF MEDICINES

C.W. Barrett, et al.
The Pharmacy Department, The London Hospital (Whitechapel),
London, E1 1BB, England

CONCLUSION

C.W. Barrett

Having described the requirements of both doctors and pharmacists that were built into the formulary preparation, I would like finally
to take two examples from the Skin Chapter to illustrate how effective
this has been.

Topical corticosteroid preparations are well known, not only
for the large number of commonly available products and their wide range
of potencies but for the extent to which they are excessively prescribed
and the pharmaceutical problems that arise in presentation, dilution and
admixtures with other active ingredients i.e. Dithranol, Coal Tar. The
formulary provides an ideal opportunity for the dermatologists and pharmacists together to eliminate all of these problems by recommending a
rational and small range of commercially available preparations, by providing concise and essential advice on their prescription and use and by
eliminating the need for subsequent dilution or admixture.

The formulary section on ulcers and pressure sores provides
another example of useful collaboration. It is still recognised that in
practice an enormous range of products are used in an attempt to treat
ulcers and pressure sores. Many of these do no good at all - some of
these do harm and most of them are unnecessarily expensive. In many cases
the doctor is not aware of what is being used and in some cases neither is
the pharmacist. Once again the formulary has provided an opportunity for
the doctor and pharmacist together to recommend simple, safe and inexpen-
sive preparations and clear cut advice.

Acknowledgement

The U.K. Organising Committee wish to thank Glaxo, ICI,
Napp and Fisons for contributions to the travelling expenses of the
U.K. teams.

RESTRICTIVE FORMULARY MANAGEMENT WITH CONSEQUENCES FOR THE
TREATMENT OF INDIVIDUAL PATIENTS

C.W.R. Phaf
Hospital pharmacist, Head department of clinical pharmacy,
St. Annadal Hospital, Maastricht, the Netherlands

As a consequence of the fact that a formulary is obligatory
the use of non-formulary drugs has to be controlled. Such control must be
exerted systematically. In daily practice this means, that every request
for a non-formulary preparation must be checked. In our department of
clinical pharmacy this is achieved by the use of a "mutation-form".

The pharmaceutical technician handling the specific request
registers on the form the following data: the name of the preparation,
the name of the patient and/or the purpose of the medication, the ward
or institution and the physician who is responsible for the request.
The technician presents the form to a pharmacist together with previous
mutation-forms for the same preparation. The pharmacist accounts for the
consideration of his consent or denial on the form. Often according to
the formulary principle the physician must be asked for the rationale of
his prescription. Furtheremore the actions taken to try and deliver the
compound and the quantities to be bought and delivered must be noted on
the mutation-form.

By consequent use of these forms we are able to follow
reasonable use and unreasonable demands of non-formulary drugs.
Conclusions may be drawn as to the quality and the managebility of a
specific formulary chapter. The data may lead to proposals to take
preparations into the formulary or to formulate specific conditions for
the use of preparations. Moreover insight in the prescribing habits of
physicians and in the treatment of individual patients may be deepened
by studying the mutation-forms over a specific period.

As a good example of formulary management we analyzed all
non-formulary requests for psychopharmaceuticals.

At the end of 1978 the formulary-principle was introduced to
the psychiatric staff. The formulary-chapters on psychopharmaceuticals

were accepted by the staff in the first half of 1979. The formulary
contains a reduced number of preparations: for instance 13 neuroleptics,
6 antidepressants, 8 benzodiazepines, sleep inducing drugs inclusive and
only lithium carbonate for lithium-therapy. It must be admitted, that
the number of preparations in the formulary might be reduced without
harming the patients but there is a bit of a compromise in any obligatory
formulary.

When the formulary committee started regulating the use of
psychopharmaceuticals we expected many problems concerning the choice of
the preparations because the psychiatric staff was not accustomed to be
subjected to any kind of audit. After all it must be recognised   that
we were dealing with a profession that claims priority to personal
argumentation and many psychologic factors. This consideration includes
physicians as well as patients.

The figures show that nevertheless regulation of psychopharmaceuticals was very well possible. The use of the mutation-sheets
to control the requests of non-formulary preparations provided a lot of
work but as the results will show it can be done and it seems to be
worth while. The analysis of the groups of psychopharmaceuticals will
deepen insight in the nature of the problems we meet.

In the period under study (1977 to 1/7-1982) we received
572 requests of non-formulary neuroleptics (62,5% of the total of psychopharmaceuticals). These requests concerned 201 patients; requested
therapy was granted for 134 patients.

The requests of phenothiazines and derivatives concerning
16 different preparations formed the majority with 478 requests (83,5%)
for 173 patients, granted for 109 patients. The therapy of 64 (37%)
patients was changed during the consultation. For the haloperidol
derivatives (haloperidol decanoate, bromperidol and one specific case
of melperon) we received 68 requests (12%), concerning 19 patients.
All requests were granted because haloperidol decanoate and bromperidol
were under study for uptake into the formulary.

Furthermore there were 26 requests for sulpiride concerning
9 patients. Most of these requests (88,5%) were delivered for 6 patients
being under this treatment since before the formulary-chapter was
introduced. The psychiatrist planned and promised to change this therapy.

The same applies to 6 patients under treatment with levomepromazine and 15 patients receiving thioproperazine, in total 155 requests.

Many requests for chlorpromazine were for use against hiccough. We advised the use of haloperidol or perphenazine. Levomepromazine was frequently requested as an adjuvant in analgesic therapy. In these cases we advise the use of haloperidol or droperidol. Most consultations concerning pain lead to an improved total regimen.

Non-formulary antidepressants were requested 71 times for 38 patients and granted for 12 patients during the period of 1979 to 1/7-1982 The preparations were nortriptyline and some non-formulary amitriptyline-forms and combination-compounds for 6 patients.

Furthermore there were 14 request for mianserin, tested by one physician for eventual uptake into the formulary.

Non-formulary requests for benzodiazepines during the period of 1978 to 1/7-1982. They concerned 101 patients. For only 39 patients the requested preparations were dispensed. One preparation under study took 45% of the total. Two other drugs were responsible for 54%. For 81% of the patients these requests were denied.

Barbiturates and hexapropimate are banned effectively. Phenobarbital is the only barbiturate used and the only indication is for some cases of epilepsy. In the period of 1978 to 1/7-1982 we received only 36 requests for 24 patients. These requests were granted for 9 patients as a start for a detoxication period.

Lithiumcarbonate is the only formulary preparation for lithium-therapy. We received 27 requests for a sustained-release preparation. Requests were granted for one patient having gastric disturbances after taking lithiumcarbonate, for one patient dependant on form and colour and for four patients to be changed to lithiumcarbonate within 3-4 weeks.

The total of requests for non-formulary psychopharmaceuticals illustrates the workload of the daily practice of the mutation forms. 916 Non-formulary requests for psychopharmaceuticals were registered in the period from 1977 to 1/7-1982. These prescriptions concerned 386 patients. The requested therapy was granted for 217 patients (56%) and denied for 169 cases (44%).

9 Preparations tested for eventual uptake into the formulary or under research for other specific purposes were responsable for 29%

of the requests (268) and concerned 20,5% of the patients(79).

A group of 37 patients were placed under a regimen of psycho-
pharmacotherapy before the formulary-chapter was proposed. Their old-
time-pharmacotherapy can be changed into an improved regimen. The one
psychiatrist who treats these patients promised to do so but until this
moment the promise had no follow-up. That means a workload of 200 requests
(22%) for this group of patients.

Another small group of problem-patients are the patients
coming from outside the hospital, who are to be detoxicated from barbiturates. We registered 7 cases.

Most other requests that were granted are due to a careful
start of formulary-policy and during the last two years they concern
patients or in some cases physicians with very specific psychological
motives.

The educative effect of the management-policy is clearly
illustrated by the discussions concerning the 152 requests for promethazine for 112 patients, granted for only 46 patients. Promethazine was
the ancestor of a long series of neuroleptics. Therefore physicians tend
to forget that it is not a neuroleptic itself. They don't acknowledge
that in the meantime we have better medication against cough, itch and
pain and that we have safer and more effective antiallergics, sedatives,
antiemetics and sleepinducers.

Based on this analysis we know that the tremendous workload
of the way we handle the exceptional requests is worth while. Especially
the observation that our call frequently triggers a consultative
discussion leading to an improved therapy regimen is an encouraging
stimulus.

CHANGES IN ANALGESIC PATTERNS

TRIQUELL LL, PARDO C, AGUSTI C, MAS M.P.
Granollers General Hospital. Pharmacy Service.
Granollers. Barcelona. Spain.

INTRODUCTION

The use of therapeutic analgesics in Spanish Hospitals differs from the standard use of analgesics in the Hospitals of Central Europe and the United States.

The main objective of this discussion is to rationalize our method in the use of analgesics at the Granollers General Hospital (GGH)

The following is an analysis of the history of analgesic prescription in 1978 and 1982 and analgesic consumption at the hospital between 1978 and 1981.

METHODOLOGY

The central difficulties in this rationalization program were:
- The existing prescription habit was very difficult to change.
- Both physicians and nurses were involved.
- Many aspects of the analgesics problem were not taken into consideration.

We approached the problem in several different ways:
1) In 1979 the P.T.C. prepared some informational bulletins and the following titles were issued:
    - Analgesic Consumption Analysis
    - Neoplastic Chronic Pain Treatment
    - Rational Analgesic Administration
    - Analgesic prescription 1st part: Salicylates and Acetaminophen revision.
    - Analgesic prescription 2nd part: Pirazolones and other non-steroid anti-inflammatory drug revision.
    - Narcotic revision.

2)   Clinical Sessions were held with the Medical Teams.

3)   Analgesic Pharmacotherapy seminaries were given for the
     nurses:
     - Recommended by the nurse station these were 10 hour
       courses, divided into two shifts so as to involve the
       largest number of Nurses possible.

4)   We estabished a new rule regarding "as required" analge-
     sic prescriptions:
     - Every "as required" prescription would be renewed
       every two (2) days.
       If it was not renewed, it would be terminated.

RESULTS AND DISCUSSION

By studying the total analgesic consumption occurring at the
Hospital between 1978 and 1981 we observe the following: (Fig. 1)
table (1   , 2)

1 - Stabilization in the use of Acetaminophen/Dextropropoxiphene

2 - Increase in the use of Acetaminophen

3 - Increase in the use of opioids consumption (Fig. 2 , 3)

4 - Strong increase in the use of Salicylates (Fig. 4)

5 - Decrease of Dipyrones consumption (Fig. 5)

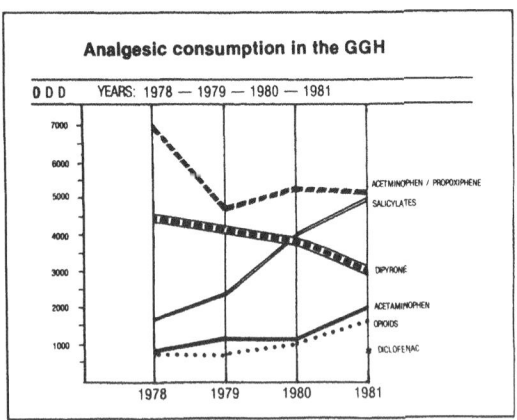

Fig. 1 : Analgesic consumption
         in the GGH(1978-1979) (1980-1981)

	1978	%	1979	%	1980	%	1981	%
DIPYRONE	4.404	30	4.096	31	3.802	24	2.955	17
SALICYLATES	1.746	12	2.382	18	4.148	26	4.941	29
ACETAMINOPHEN	820	6	1.192	9	1.093	7	1.956	12
ACETAMINOPHEN PROPOXIPHENE	6.825	47	4.710	36	5.530	35	5.402	32
DICLOFENAC							710	2
PENTAZOCINE	390	2	379	3	533	3	848	5
MEPERIDINE	416	3	308	2	338	2	492	3
MORPHINE	6	0,04	83	0,5	139	1	158	1
	14.607		13.150		15.682		16.989	
BROMPTON'S MIXTURE			529		612		2.060	

Table I.   DDD analgesics used in the GGH. 1978-1979-1980-1981

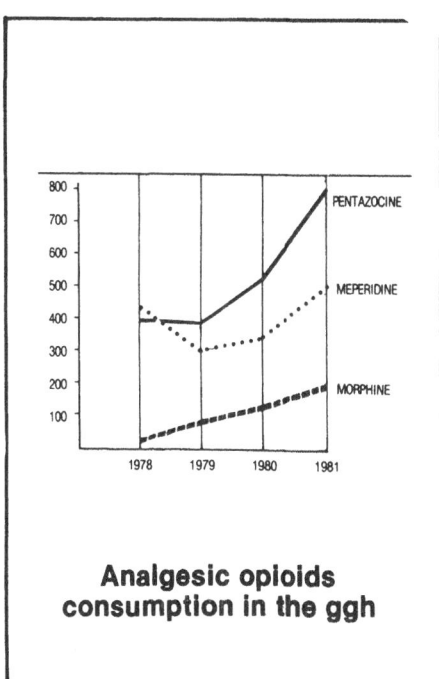

**Analgesic opioids
consumption in the ggh**

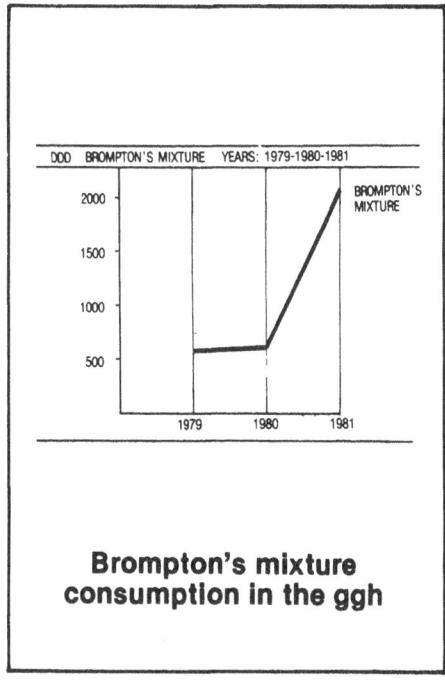

**Brompton's mixture
consumption in the ggh**

Fig. 2   Analgesic opioids
         consumption in the GGH

Fig. 3   Brompton's mixture
         consumption in the GGH

ANALGESIC	D D D	1978	1979	1980	1981
Acetylsalicylic Acid	3 g	390	584	1.214	1.265
Microencapsulated Acetylsalicylic Acid	3 g	146	169	160	470
Acetylsalicylic Acid TOTAL		536	753	1.374	1.735
Lysine Acetylsalicylate oral	3 g	998	1.364	2.157	2.138
Lysine Acetylsalicylate parenteral	3 g	212	265	616	1.068
Lysine Acetylsalicylate TOTAL		1.210	1.629	2.773	3.206
Acetaminophen Dextropropoxyphene	3 cáps.	6.825	4.710	5.530	5.402
Acetaminophen Butalbital Codeine	4 cáps.	479	522	422	313
Cibalgina® supos.	4 supos	331	287	273	--
Acetaminophen oral	2 g	35	215	260	843
Acetaminophen rectal	2 g	306	455	411	800
Acetaminophen TOTAL		341	670	671	1.643
Dipyrone amp.	6 g	1.464	1.242	1.172	843
Dipyrone supos	3 g	307	298	281	161
Dipyrone TOTAL		1.771	1.540	1.453	1.004
Baralgin® amp.	3 amp.	1.700	1.667	1.484	1.772
Baralgin® supos	3 supos	120	--	--	179
Baralgin® TOTAL		1.820	1.667	1.484	1.951
Buscapina Compositum amp.	3 amp.	436	576	524	--
Buscapina Compositum supos	3 supos	46	26	68	--
Buscapina Compositum TOTAL		482	602	592	--
Pentazocine amp.	0,2 g	390	379	533	848
Meperidine amp.	0,24 g	416	308	338	492
Mophine amp.	30 mg	6	83	139	158
Methadone amp.	25 mg	--	--	--	10

Table II.   DDD used in the GGH. 1978-1979-1980-1981.

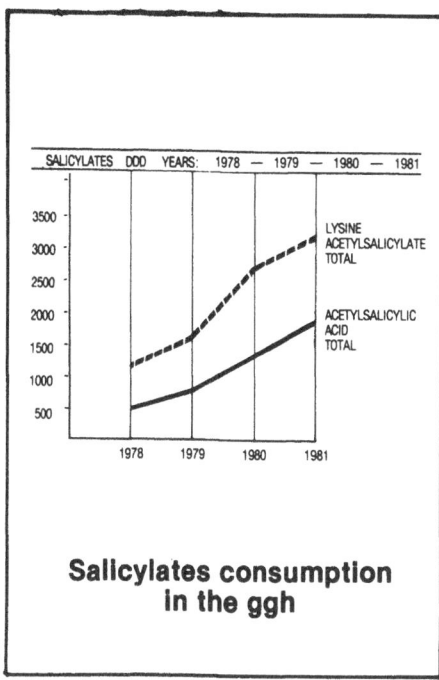

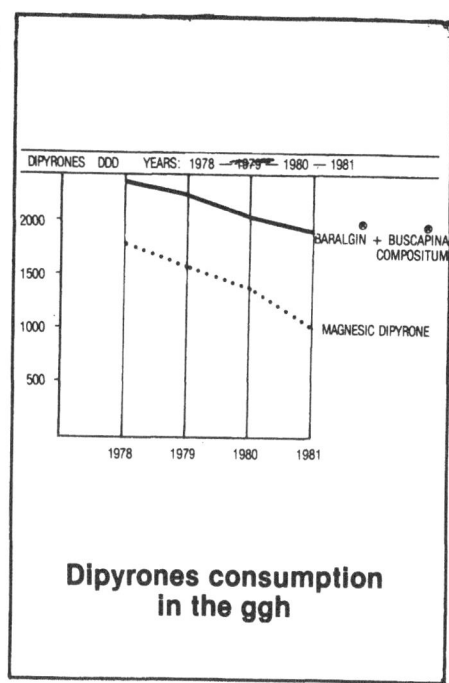

-Fig. 4 Salicylates consumption   Fig. 5 Dipyrones consumption
          in the GGH   in the GGH

        The results of a study we made of the years 1978 and 1982
of the analgesic prescription in the Medical Services are shown in
Fig (6, 7)

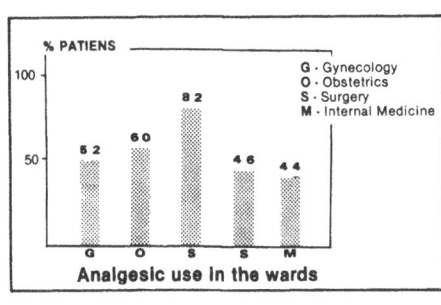

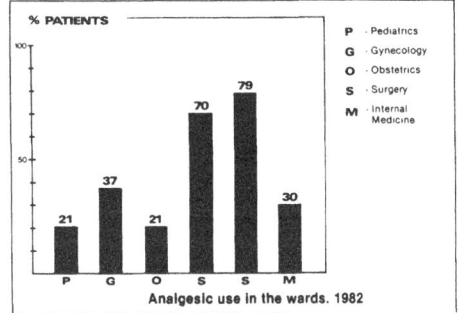

Fig. 6 Analgesic use in the   Fig. 7 Analgesic use in the
         wards 1978   wards 1982

The study of "as required" analgesics prescription rate is shown in Fig. (8 , 9)

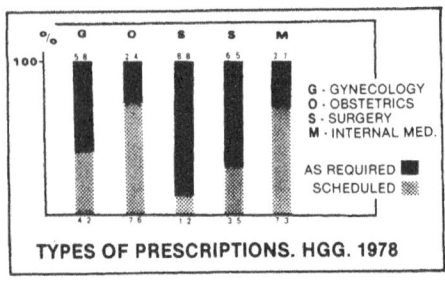

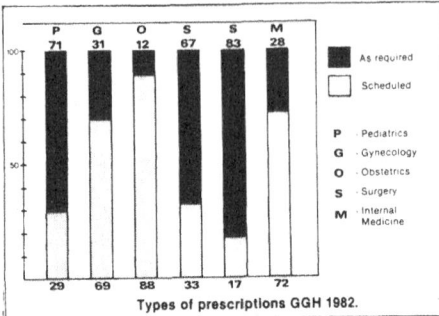

Fig. 8   Types of prescriptions   Fig. 9   Types of prescriptions
        GGH 1978   GGH 1982

Here we note that the hours of administration for the " as required" analgesics are almost identical for both periods of time. This is a consequence of having an excessive rate of "as required" prescriptions which were very difficult to change. Fig. (10 , 11)

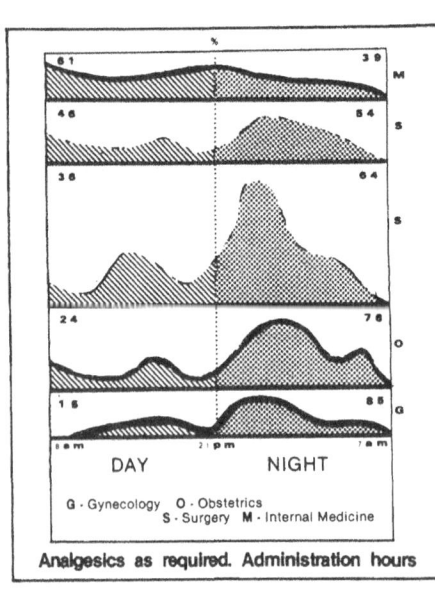

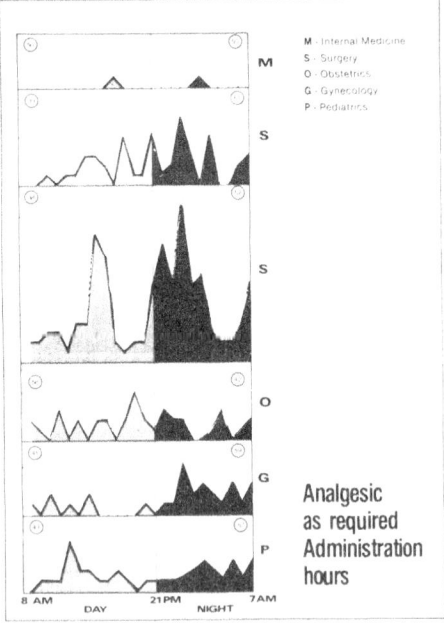

Fig. 10   Analgesics as required   Fig. 11 Analgesics as required
        Administration hours 1978   Administration hours 1982

CONCLUSIONS

We offered some alternatives to the spasmolitic associated dipyrones and have been successful in finding suitable replacements. By steady lowering the rate of use of Dipyrones we will eventually be able to remove them from the Formulary altogether.

We will try to modify the high index of oral ASL by orientating the hospital staff towards the use of Salicylates.

" As required" analgesic is another point we must act upon in view of the fact that there was no change in its prescription incidence, even when a rule was established.

Buscapina Compositum®: Scopolamine butyl bromide, Sodium Noramidopyrine Methanesulphonate.

Baralgin® : Sodium Noramidopyrine. Methanesulphonate, 4' (beta-piperidinoetoxi) carbo- (2)- methoxi-benzophenone, Fenpipramide Hcl.

CLINICAL PHARMACY IMPROVEMENT AND INTERRELATION WITH THERAPEUTIC TEAM

PARDO, C. MAS, M.P. AGUSTI, C. TRIQUELL, LL
Granollers General Hospital. Pharmacy Service. Granollers
Barcelona. Spain.

INTRODUCTION

Since the mid 1960s pharmacists practicing in hospitals have taken an active role in developing new pharmaceutical services directed toward reducing problems associated with drug use. This movement was born in the USA and gradually has spread to the European Countries.

The entity of Clinical Pharmacy has been clearly defined (OSTINO 1980) (Fig. 1)

1	DRUG DISTRIBUTION (UNIT-DOSE)
2	IV. PARENTERAL ADMIXTURE
3	TOTAL AND ENTERAL NUTRITION PROCEDURES
4	DRUG MANUFACTURING AND CONTROL
5	DRUG INFORMATION
6	THERAPEUTIC HOSPITAL FORMULARY MANAGEMENT
7	MEDICATION HISTORY AND THERAPEUTIC PROFILE
8	IN AND OUT-PATIENTS COUNSELLING
9	CLINICAL PHARMACOKINETIC SERVICE
10	DRUG UTILISATION REVIEW PROGRAMS

Figure 1. Clinical Pharmacy ideal profile.

One of the most important problems of this entity is the differences that exist between countries when they apply the Clinical Pharmacy Programs.

When a Clinical Pharmacy Program is introduced in the Hospital, independently of its complexity, it must be evaluated. Like in other areas of konwledge the effectiveness of the introduced program must be realized. (LEACH 1981, PATHAC 1981).

Until now in the Pharmaceutical Service of the Granollers General Hospital (G.G.H.), when we tried to evaluate the effectiveness of our clinical activity we studied defined situations of pharmacological therapeutics like: Analgesics (TRIQUELL, LL 1980) Antibiotics, fluids and electrolytes (PARDO, C 1981).

Our aim is to study clinical functions of the Pharmaceutical Service in collaboration with the Hospital's Medical Services and discern the acceptance of the pharmacist's contribution by physicians and nurses.

METHODOLOGY

The Granollers General Hospital (G.G.H.) is a 227 bed non-profit hospital. The pharmaceutical service was created in 1973. The present staff in composed of three staff pharmacists and one assistant pharmacist.

Since 1974 we have used a unit dose drug distribution system (UDDDS). Now it applies to the whole hospital. The hospital expenditures for drugs in 1981 were $ 235,000

The pharmaceutical clinical activity has been evaluated by counting the number of contributions in therapeutic matters in which a pharmacist has taken part. Two kinds of contributions have been assessed: ACTIVE and PASSIVE CONTRIBUTIONS, in the first case the pharmacist has taken the initiative , in the second a therapeutic question has been made to him. In both cases the pharmacist has come in contact with physicians and nurses.

Active contributions were performed by using the UDDDS as an essential base. Analysing and recording the physician's prescriptions are the informative sources to come in contact personal or by telephone with physicians and/or the nurses. In our hospital two staff pharmacists carry out this function. They look after a fixed number of beds an take care of all the pharmaceutical problems which those patients can generate. In order to control the treatment duration, a special form has been used. With it the physician knows how long a drug has been used, and reminds him of the need to make a new prescription.

Another aspect is drug monitoring. Since our hospital cannot do pharmacokinetic control of the drugs used, a strict control over drugs was performed. (Fig. 2)

DRUGS/PATIENTS	COLOUR	POSITION
ANTIBIOTICS	BLUE	1
ORAL ANTICOAGULANTS	RED	3
NARCOTIC DRUGS	GREEN	5
DIGOXIN	WHITE	7
THEOPHYLLINE	BROWN	9
OTHERS	BLACK	11
PATIENTS TAKING MORE THAN 7 DRUGS AT THE SAME TIME	BLACK	29-30
PATIENTS WITH PHARMACIST CONTRIBUTION	VIOLET	26

Figure 2. Drugs and patients monitored

In order to find patients with a certain drug treatment easily our old pharmacotherapeutic profile was adapted. We began to use coloured signs to see the profile of either patients or drug treatments and achieve a better control. (Fig. 3) We use the " observation section " of pharmacotherapeutic profile to record the contribution which has been performed. When a patient is discharged from the hospital, a clinical session is made in the Pharmacy Service where all the staff discuss and evaluate the contribution performed.

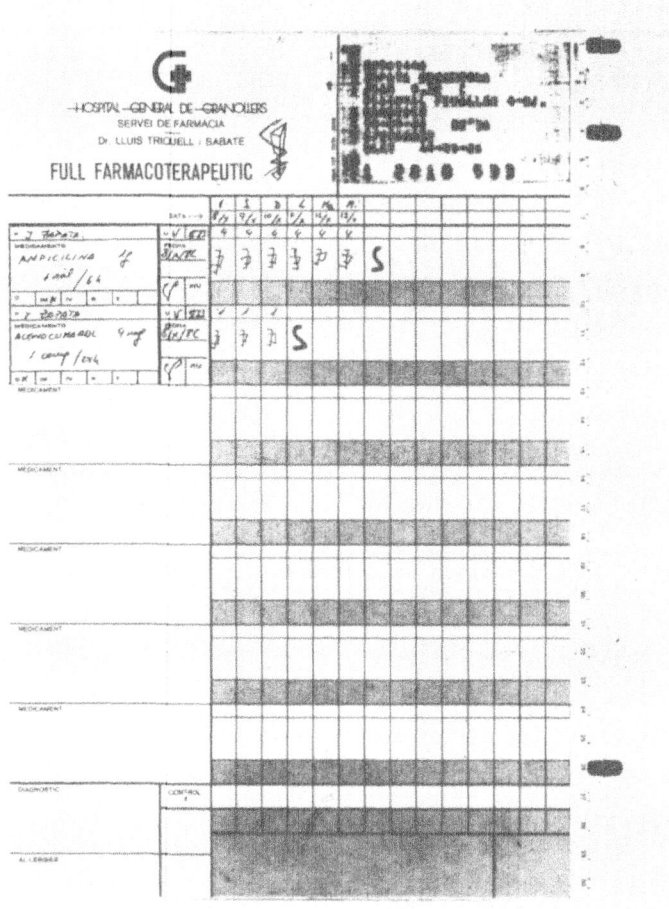

Figure 3. Pharmacotherapeutic profile of G.G.H.

RESULTS AND DISCUSSION

The Period studied is ten weeks long from 1/4/82 to 15/6/82 During this period of time 2,395 patients were hospitalized. The Pharmacy Service made 108 contributions in 96 patients (4% of the hospitalized patients). Table 1   shows the distribution of the Pharmaceutical Service's contributions based on the Medical Service where this contributions were made.

MEDICAL SERVICE	NUMBER OF CONTRIBUTIONS	ACTIVE CONTRIBUTIONS	PASSIVE CONTRIBUTIONS
INTERNAL MEDICINE	26	15 (58%)	11 (42%)
SURGERY	32	32 (100%)	0 (0%)
OBSTETRICS-GYNECOLOGY	44	40 (91%)	4 (9%)
PEDIATRICS	5	2 (40%)	3 (6o%)
OTHERS	1	0 (0%)	1 (100%)
TOTAL	108	89 (82%)	19 (18%)

Table 1. Distribution of pharmacist collaboration with
Medical Services in the G.G.H.

Pharmaceutical Service profile of contributions are different
accoding to the Medical Services. While passive contributions in Internal Medicine and Pediatrics are an elevated percentage passive contributions in the Surgery, Obstetrics and Gynecology Services are almost
negligible.

We think that the ideal profile of contributions would be
similar to the Internal Medicine one, because it is the result of the
close collaboration that we want to extend to the other services of the
Hospital.

Table 2 shows the drugs which we have contributed. We must
emphasize some groups of drugs like antibiotics and analgesics. These
groups of drugs are areas of great interest in the Pharmaceutical Service
because of their economic mass and their therapeutic importance. The Pharmaceutical Service has been collaborating with other Services on these
therapeutic areas for some years. In the other groups of drugs, Theophylline, Cimetidine, Corticosteroids, Heparin, Acenocoumarol, and Parenteral/
Enteral Nutrition are responsible for most of the contributions.

The spectrum of contributions which has been carried out over
pharmacological therapeutics is shown in table 3 and 4

ANTIBIOTICS	n°
AMPICILLIN ------------------	28
GENTAMICIN ------------------	18
PENICILLIN G PROCAINE -------	4
CEPHALOSPORINS --------------	3
CO-TRIMOXAZOLE --------------	2
LINCOMYCIN ------------------	2
NALIDIXIC ACID --------------	2
NITROFURANTOIN --------------	1
STREPTOMYCIN ----------------	1
RIFAMPIN --------------------	1
ISONIAZID -------------------	1
ETHAMBUTOL ------------------	1
COLIMYCIN -------------------	1
SULPHASALAZINE --------------	1
TOTAL ---	66

ANALGESICS	n°
PENTAZOCINE ----------------	12
LYSINE ACETYLSALICYLATE ----	3
PARACETAMOL DEXTROPROPOXYPHENE ---------	2
CODEINE --------------------	1
DICLOFENAC -----------------	1
MAGNESIUM DIPYRONE ---------	1
BENORILATE -----------------	1
OXYPHENBUTAZONE ------------	1
BROMPTON'S MIXTURE ---------	1
ANTI-INFLAMMATORY AGENTS ---	1
TOTAL --	24

VITAMINS AND MINERALS	n°
VITAMIN C ------------------	3
VITAMIN D ------------------	2
CALCIUM --------------------	2
VITAMIN B COMPLEX ----------	1
TOTAL --	8

GASTROINTESTINAL DRUG	n°
METOCLOPRAMIDE ------------	2
BISACODYL -----------------	2
MAGNESIUM SULPHATE --------	2
ALUMINUM PHOSPHATE --------	2
DIPHENOXYLATE -------------	1
TOTAL ---	9

OTHERS	
THEOPHYLLINE --------------	4
CIMETIDINE ----------------	2
HEPARIN -------------------	2
ACENOCOUMAROL -------------	1
DIGOXIN -------------------	1
CHLORMETHIAZOLE -----------	1
HYDROCHLOROTHIAZIDE -------	1
CHLORHEXIDINE -------------	1
HEXETIDINE ----------------	1
ACETYLCYSTEINE ------------	1
DIETHYLSTILBESTROL --------	1
TESTOSTERONE --------------	1
D-CHLORPHENIRAMINE --------	1
PARENTERAL NUTRITION-------	1
ENTERAL NUTRITION ---------	2
HYPNOTICS -----------------	1
CORTICOSTEROIDS -----------	2
STREPTOKINASE/ STREPTODORNASE ------------	1
MODECATE® ----------------	1
TOTAL --	26

Table 2. Drugs implicated in Pharmaceutical contributions

CONTRIBUTIONS	n°	%
DURATION OF DRUG TREATMENT	49	56
CHOICE OF DRUG TREATMENT	18	21
DOUBLE DRUG TREATMENT	11	13
DRUGS NON ADMINISTERED	4	5
DOSIFICATION	3	3
DRUG ADMINISTRATION METHODS	1	1
CHOICE OF DOSAGE FORMS	1	1
TOTAL	87	100

Table 3.   Active contributions studied in the G.G.H.

CONTRIBUTIONS	n°	%
CHOICE OF DRUG TREATMENT	14	66
DOSIFICATION	4	19
TOXICOLOGICAL INFORMATION	1	5
DRUG INTERATIONS INFORMATION	1	5
SIDE EFFECTS OF DRUGS INFORMATION	1	5
TOTAL	21	100

Table 4.   Passive contributions studied in G.G.H.

We have differentiated between passive and active contributions.

When we studied active contributions " Duration of a drug
treatment " was the subject discussed the most, leading to 49 contributions. Most of them were due to antibiotics treatments (33 contributions)
and analgesic treatments (11 contributions), the other two contributions
involved other pharmacological groups.

There are some points which differentiate the spectrum of
passive and active contributions, for example, "drug administration methods" and "choice of dosage forms". Both appear in the spectrum

without being in the passive one

" Choice of drug treatment" and "Drug dosification" are
common in both profiles of contributions.

The clinical contributions were evaluated by the Pharmaceutical Service Staff. A contribution was considered   positive if the
pharmaceutical point of view was taken in to account by the physician.
When the contrary took place, it was considered a negative contribution.
And finally it was an indifferent contribution when there was no opportunity of verifying its result for example when a patient was discharged
from the Hospital. Results are shown in table 5. The acceptance we have
now reached is high, 85% of total contributions.

EVALUATION OF CONTRIBUTIONS	n°	%
POSITIVE	92	85
NEGATIVE	7	6
INDIFFERENT	9	9
TOTAL	100	100

Table 5. Evaluation of pharmaceutical contribution in
the G.G.H.

CONCLUSIONS

The need for clinical activity evaluation is an evident fact
that we have verified with our experience. The benefits of the evaluation
will become clear it its conclusions serve to establish mechanisms which
help to improve the activities of the Clinical Pharmacy programs.

In this study there is a tendency of no collaboration in
Pediatrics which perhaps needs a change in our attitude.

Likewise, Obstetrics-Gynecology and Surgery Services didn't
collaborated at the same rate as Internal Medicine. It's necesary for
us to analyze why this is so, and correct our approach.

This experience has pushed us to initiate more specific
evaluation systems by developing new collaboration forms. It will
gradually improve our possibilities in the Clinical Pharmacy exercise.

REFERENCES:

LEACH, R.H., et al (1981). An evaluation of ward pharmacy service. Journal of Clinical and Hospital Pharmacy 6 : 173-182

OSTINO, G (1980) General Practice on Clinical Pharmacy. In Aulagner, G. Plasse, J.C. ,Van der klein, E. Progress in Clinical Pharmacy II, Amsterdam,   Elsevier/North Holland Biomedical Press (1980) 3-11

PARDO, C. et al (1981) Evaluation of intravenous therapy criteria in the General Hospital of Granollers. 10th European Symposium on Clinical Pharmacy Stresa. Italy.

PATHAC S (1981) Evaluation of Clinical Programs: an operational Frame work. Drug Intelligence an Clinical Pharmacy 15: 459-468

TRIQUELL, LL. et al (1980) Analgesic in Clinical Practice: Drug use review. Aulagner, G. Plasse, J.C., Van der Klein, E. Progress in Clinical Pharmacy II, Amsterdam.   Elsevier/North Holland Biomedical Press : 43-53

CLINICAL PHARMACIST PARTICIPATION IN A CLINICAL
TRIAL - TREATMENT OF CONGESTIVE HEART FAILLURE

M.A. SOARES

A.C. GONÇALVES

R.M. SANTOS

V.M. RAMALHINHO

L. RAVARA

Department of Pharmacy - University Hospital of
St. Maria,
1292 LISBOA CODEX - PORTUGAL

Patients in Congestive Heart Failure (CHF) resistan
t ·to conventional treatment of digitalis and diuretics fre -
quently attend our hospital. Backed by the works of Opie, Bar
ry with vasodilators we also have tried to get an increase of
left ventricular performance in these patients.

We elaborated a protocol using Isosorbide Dinitrate
(ISDN) alone or in combination with Hydralazine associated to
the digitalis and diuretics. The study is a double blind one
and the patients were randomly allocated in two groups. Both
are medicated with digoxin 0.25 mg once daily, furosemide
40 mg twice daily and isosorbide dinitrate 30 mg three times
daily. One of the groups was on placebo and the other group

P R O T O C O L

A GROUP	Digoxin	-	0.25 mg once daily
	Furosemide	-	40 mg b.i.d.
	ISDN	-	30 mg t.i.d.
	Placebo	-	twice daily
B GROUP	Digoxin	-	0.25 mg once daily
	Furosemide	-	40 mg b.i.d.
	ISDN	-	30 mg t.i.d.
	Hydralazine	-	50 mg b.i.d.

Table 1

was on hydralazine 50 mg twice daily (Table 1).

The patients are monitorized according to the clinical and laboratory   parameters, namely: electrocardiogram,
chest X-Ray, heart rate, blood pressure, diuresis, weight and
plasma levels of urea, creatinine, ionogram and liver func -
tions tests. They are classified according to the New York
Heart Association (NYHA) before the treatment and at the moment they left the hospital. All were submited to an echocar-
diogram to assess roughly left ventricular performance.

As one of the vasodilators we choose isosorbide dini
trate in high oral doses as a result of its known pharmacological effects and its pharmacokinetics properties. In B group
we added hydralazine, an arteriolar vasodilator trying to assess if we could upgrade the results obtained in A group with
ISDN alone.

Isosorbide dinitrate in patients with heart failure
seems to have some different cardiovascular effects from those observed in healthy ones. This is a vasodilator with seg-
mental and regional differences, so it determines a strong
vasodilatation of the major post-capillary capacity vessels,
which is most apparent in healthy vascular regions, hence a
decrease in preload, neutralizing the high peripheric vascular resistence, which exists in patients with heart failure,
as stated by Ross. This reduction determines an increase of
ejection fraction, stroke volume, cardiac output and tissue
perfusion, reducing the pulmonary and peripheric edema.

Isosorbide dinitrate is rapidly and totally absorbed
by the oral route, but the drug suffers an effect of first-
-pass by the liver, reducing the bioavailability. Although
the plasma level of the sublingually administered isosorbide
dinitrate is twice as high as that of the orally administered,
this disadvantage can be offset by a higher oral dose, special
ly as there is a linear relationship between the administered
dose and the plasma concentration reached. The half-life of
ISDN, by oral route is about 1/2 h. It is metabolized via glu

tathion-organic nitrate reductase in two denitrated compounds,
5-isosorbide mononitrate (5-ISMN) with an half-life of 2.5
hours and 2-isosorbide mononitrate (2-ISMN) with an half-life
of 2.8 hours. The two mononitrates are active as vasodilators
although their potencies are weaker than the parent compound.
These metabolites are glucoronated and excreted 80-100 per
cent in 24 hours by the kidney.

We admitted until now ten male patients with their
ages between 48-78 years old (mean age 65.9). Congestive
Heart Failure of our patients was attributable to several
causes, but the principal one was cardiomyopathy in 6 patients, aortic stenosis in one and pulmonary embolism in another
patient. Five were in class III and five in class IV of NYHA.
The patients eligible to the study were randomly allocated to
their inscription number attributed prior to their attendance
in the general emergency room at our hospital. Those with even
number were included in A group (7) and the odd number were
in B group (3).(Table 2).

PRESENTATION OF THE PATIENTS IN THE STUDY UNTIL NOW

```
Number ———    10

Sex     ———    male

Age (years)-   48 - 78 (mean 65.9)

                    (Cardiomyopathy      - 6
                    )Hipertension        - 2
Etiology of CHF )Aortic stenosis        - 1
                    )Pulmonary embolism  - 1

Classification (NYHA) (Class III - 5
                       )Class  IV - 5

NQ of patients of the groups (A - 7
                              )B - 3
```

Table 2

The mean duration of the stay in the hospital was 19 days in A group with 1 death   and 16 days in B group, with two deaths.   No important side effects, and none of the pa- tients had to stop therapy as result of unwanted effects (Table 3).

RESULTS OF THE TREATMENT OF CHF (I)

Duration of the treatment- $\begin{cases} \text{A group - 19 days (1 decease)} \\ \text{B group - 16 days (2 deceases)} \end{cases}$

Important side effects   -   None

Number of deaths   - $\begin{cases} \text{A group - 1 patient} \\ \text{B group - 2 patients} \end{cases}$

Table 3

Both of the groups lost weight during the treatment, mean value of decrease of weight was 4.8 Kg to the A group and and 1 Kg to the B group. The diurese per day was in mean value of 1760 ml to A group and 900 ml to B group. The majority of the patients presented a small fall in mean blood pressure, as stated in slides. Only two patients presented an increase of 15 mm Hg in the systolic blood pressure and one of them presented an increase of the diastolic blood pressure from 40 to 90 mm Hg and the other patient maintained his value. In A group there was a mean decrease of heart rate of 18 beats per minute in 4 patients and an increase of 5 b.p.m. in 3 patients. In B group the only survivor presented a de - crease of 10 b.p.m. in heart rate (Figure 1).

RESULTS OF THE STUDY (II)

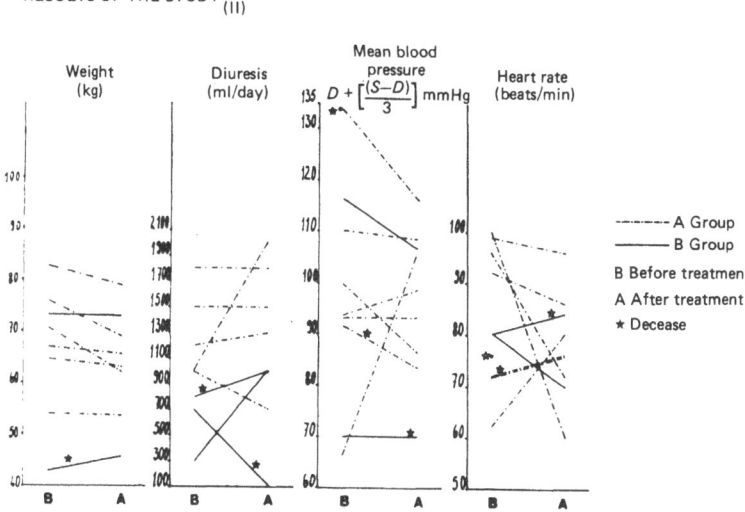

Figure 1

Minor variations of plasma levels of urea, creatini
ne, ionogram and liver function tests were recorded.

The chest X-Ray shows a decrease of cardiothoracic-
-ratio in 3 patients of A group and in the survivor of B
group. Pleural effusion and hilar accentuation were reduced
in majority of the patients who presented it.(Table 4).

RESULTS OF THE TREATMENT OF CHF (IV)

	Cardiothoracic ratio		Pleural effusion		Hilar accentuation	
	Tol.	Red.	Tot.	Red.	Tot.	Red.
A Group	7	3	3	3	3	2
B Group	3	1	2	1	1	1

TABLE 4

There was no alterations in the E.C.G. except in 2 patients of A group. One presented an improvement of the ventricular repolarization and reduction of the number of supraventricular premature beats. The other showed a reduction of the degree of atrioventricular block.

The final classification in NYHA classes was as follows: class I three patients, class II three patients and one decrease in the A group; in the B group, the one survivor was classified in the class II and two of the patients died during the study, although one of them had a sudden death when he was in class II of the NYHA (Table 5).

ALTERATIONS IN THE NYHA CLASSIFICATION

	Bef. Treatment		With Vasodilators		Nº
	Class III	Class IV	Class II	Class I	Deaths
A Group	3	4	3	3	1
B Group	2	1	1	-	2

Table 5

This preliminary report of our study still includes a very small number of patients in order to obtain any statis tical results. As stated by others we find very useful the addition of vasodilators to conventional therapy.

Isosorbide dinitrate seems to be a good choice and its addition to Hydralazine didn't upgrade the results of ISDN alone in this limited number of patients, perhaps as a result of the low dose used in the protocol.

References

- Assinder, D.F.et al. (1977). Plasma Isosorbide Dinitrate concentration in Human Subjects after administration of standart and sustained-release formulations. Journal of Ph. Sciences. Vol. 66, Nº 6, June, 775-8.

- Barry, et al (1981). Long-term vasodilators therapy for Heart Failure: Clinical response and its relationship to Hemodynamic measurements . Circulation, 63, Nº 2, 269-78.

- Down, W.H. et al. (1974). Biotransformation of Isosorbide Dinitrate in Humans. Journal of Ph. Sciences, Vol. 63, Nº 7, July, 1147-49.

- Elkajan, V. et al. (1982). Glyceryl Trinitrate (Nitroglycerin) Ointment and Isosorbide Dinitrate: A review of their Pharmacological Properties and Therapeutic Use. Drugs 23:165-94.

- Goldstein, R.E. et al. (1971). Clinical and Circulatory effects of Isosorbide Dinitrate. Circulation. Vol. 63, May, 629-40.

- Medical Letter (The), (1978). Vol. 20, Nº 20, 6 October, 89-91.

- Needleman, P. et al. (1980). Vasodilators and the treatment of angine. Pharmacological Basis of Therapeutics, 6th edition, 819-27.

- Opie , L.H. (1980). Vasodilators Drugs: The Lancet, 3 May, 966-72.

- Opie , L.H. (1980). Which drug for which disease . The Lancet, 10 May, 1012-17

- Orr, J.M. et al. (1978). Plasma concentrations of Isosorbide Dinitrate and two major metabolites following oral administration of two formulations of Isosorbide Dinitrate tablets. Can. J. of Pharm. Sciences. Vol. 13, Nº 2, 45-7.

Packer, M. (1982). Selection of vasodilators drugs for patients with severe chronic heart failure: an approach based an a New Classification. Drugs 24:64-74.

Schneider , W. et al (1981). German Detsch. Arztblatt, 12, 563-70.

Walsh. W.F. et al (1981). Results of long-term vasodilator therapy in patients with refractory congestive heart failure. Circulation, Vol. 64. Nº 3, 499-505.

Williams et al (1977). Am. J. of Cardiology, Vol.39, Jan. 84-90.

METRONIDAZOLE PLASMA LEVELS AFTER I.V. AND RECTAL ADMINISTRATION

Mangues,M.A.; Pujol,F. and Bonal,J.
Hospital de la Santa Creu i Sant Pau. Pharmacy
Service. Barcelona. Spain.

Clinically, Metronidazole is as effective as
Clindamycin against anaerobes (Stranz & Bradley 1981)
Metronidazole has been widely and succesfully used
for prophylaxis and treatment of anaerobic infections, and
some clinical trials have demonstrated the efficacy of
suppositories formulations (Goulton 1978; Foster 1981).
Metronidazole is commercially available for I.V.
administration and in tablets for oral and vaginal use. I.V.
preparation is very expensive and it was the only alternative
to oral tablets when the oral administration was not
advisable.
In 1981 a paper appeared in New Engl. J. Med.
(Ioannides et al. 1981) showing that rectal administration of
Metronidazole in suppositories gave plasma levels of the drug
quite similar to I.V. administration. This fact moved us to
perfom a similar study. The main difference between our
study and Ioannides one is that we have performed it
according with the prophylactic protocol of our Hospital.

MATERIALS AND METHODS

Sixteen patients from the G.I. Surgery Service of
our Hospital that underwent gastrectomy or rectal or colon
surgery were admitted for the study. They ranged in age from
46 to 81 years and in weight from 45.5 to 78.6 Kg. Patients
suffering from diarrheic diseases were excluded for rectal
administration of Metronidazole and no patient had hepatic
failure. Concomitant therapy with barbiturates, rifampicin

and phenytoin was also a reason of exclusion.

Three dosage forms were compared:

I.V. solution: Metronidazole 500 mg in 100 ml (Flagyl[R] injectable,Rhône-Poulenc Farma, S.A.E.).

Suppository: Metronidazole 500 mg and 750 mg in Estearinum base A and B.

Enema: Metronidazole 500 mg and 750 mg in arabic gum 10% solution. The suppositories and the enemas were compounded in our Pharmacy Service.

Five groups of patients were established according to the route of administration and dose. Table 1 shows them.

All patients received three doses of Metronidazole at 8 hours intervals. The first one was administered 2 hours before surgery. One blood sample was drawn immediately before the second dose administration (at time zero). Further samples were taken at prefixed intervals before the third dose.

Plasma concentrations of Metronidazole were determined by high pressure liquid chromatography. (Marques 1978).

TABLE 1. ROUTE OF ADMINISTRATION, DOSAGE FORM, DOSE AND PATIENT DATA.

ROUTE	DOSAGE FORM	DOSE (MG)	PATIENT INITIALS	SEX	AGE (YEARS)	WEIGHT (KG)
I.V.	SOLUTION	500	JCP	M	46	74.6
			MTP	M	59	78.6
			FCR	M	63	60.0
			PCN	F	74	68.5
			VBA	M	71	50.9
R	SUPPOSITORY	500	AVM	F	60	51.0
E			DPS	F	77	4.0
C			MGV	F	74	49.0
T			HCG	F	64	57.0
A			ERS	F	80	45.5
L		750	MQE	F	81	60.8
			RPG	F	52	50.5
			ARP	F	60	51.5
	ENEMA	500	MBC	F	65	46.2
			CCC	M	56	67.5
		750	GMV	M	61	53.0

RESULTS

Figure 1 shows the mean ± SEM of Metronidazole plasma concentrations after the second dose of rectal suppository, rectal enema and intravenous infusion.

It was calculated the area under the plasma level--time curve (AUC) for each patient. Normalized areas (AUC/Wt//D) were also obtained (Table 2).

The results from rectal suppositories and I.V. solution have been statistically analyzed. We could not perform statistical calculations of the enema results because

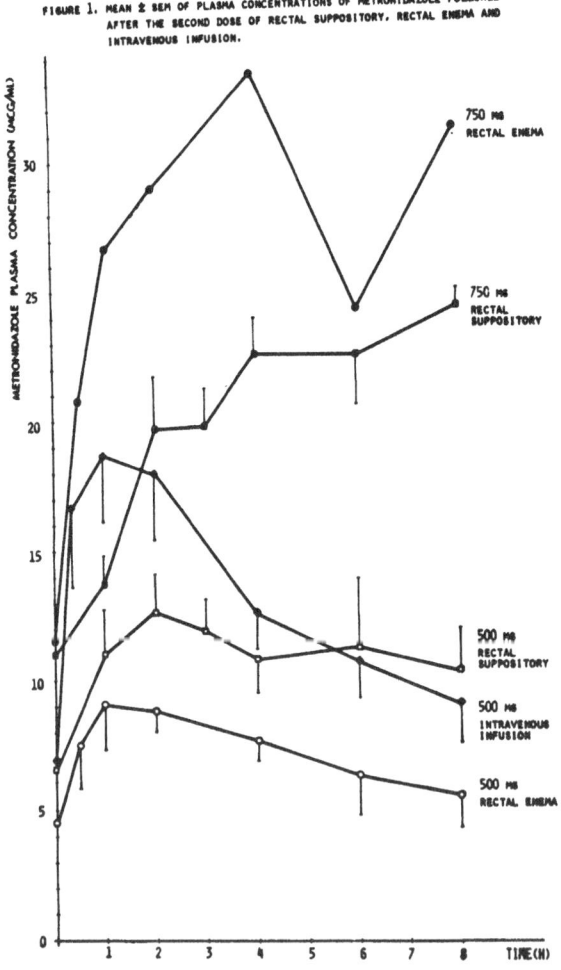

FIGURE 1. MEAN ± SEM OF PLASMA CONCENTRATIONS OF METRONIDAZOLE FOLLOWED AFTER THE SECOND DOSE OF RECTAL SUPPOSITORY, RECTAL ENEMA AND INTRAVENOUS INFUSION.

the small number of cases included in the study.

A nonparametric analysis of variance (Kruskal-
-Wallis test and test U of Mann-Whitney) was performed with
the AUC/Wt values (Siegel 1956). The results are showed in
Table 3.

Differences statistically significant were not
found between the AUC/Wt value for I.V. solution 500 mg and
rectal suppository 500 mg.

These differences were significant comparing I.V.
solution 500 mg and rectal suppository 750 mg and also
comparing the two suppositories doses (500 and 750 mg).

There were no significant differences between the
AUC/Wt/D values obtained for I.V. solution and rectal
suppositories (500 and 750 mg) neither between the initial
concentration normalized (C_i/Wt/D) obtained for the same
dosage forms. (Table 2).

The percentage of time that the plasma
concentrations of Metronidazole were kept above the minimum
inhibitory concentration (MIC= 6.2 mcg ml^{-1}) was calculated
for each group of patients (Table 4).

TABLE 2. AREAS UNDER THE PLASMA LEVEL-TIME (AUC) OBTAINED.
NORMALIZED AREAS WITH WEIGHT(AUC/ Wt) AND WEIGHT
AND DOSE (AUC/Wt/D) AND INITIAL CONCENTRATIONS
NORMALIZED (C_i/Wt/D).

		PATIENT	AUC	AUC/Wt	AUC/Wt/D	C_i/Wt/D
I.V. SOLUTION	0.5g	JCP	75.37	1.01	2.02	0.12
		MTP	96.62	1.23	2.46	0.19
		FCR	89.10	1.48	2.97	0.22
		PCN	129.16	1.89	3.77	0.18
		VBA	148.30	2.92	5.83	0.36
SUPPOSITORY	0.5g	AVM	58.40	1.15	2.29	0.16
		DPS	108.45	1.70	3.39	0.26
		MGV	84.20	1.72	3.44	0.28
		HCG	72.35	1.27	2.54	0.20
		ERS	114.70	2.52	5.04	0.35
	0.75g	MOE	140.15	2.19	2.92	0.21
		RPG	173.71	3.44	4.59	0.30
		ARP	176.60	3.46	4.62	0.32
ENEMA	0.5g	MBS	56.60	1.23	2.45	0.24
		CCC	60.55	0.89	1.79	0.11
	0.75g	CMV	234.40	2.95	5.89	0.29

Figure 2 shows the plasma concentrations of
Metronidazole after the second dose of 500 mg rectal
suppository. The mean value of maximal concentration was
reached after 2.9 hours (range 1.5 to 6 hours). Kabela et al.
(1981) found for this parameter a similar value.

DISCUSSION

This trial was designed to compare the plasma
concentrations of Metronidazole reached after I.V. and
rectal administration during the prophylactic treatment of
the patients for G.I. surgery.

When the normalized AUC (AUC/Wt) was compared for
500 mg I.V. solution and 750 mg rectal suppositories a value
of $p < 0.05$ was found. The same probability was obtained
comparing the two doses of rectal suppositories (500 and
750 mg). That means there are differences statistically
significant between these dosage forms. The AUC for the
750 mg dose is bigger than for the 500 mg dose, as can be
seen in Figure 1.

In contrast there is no difference between the
I.V. solution (500 mg) and the rectal suppository (500 mg)
neither between all the dosage forms when the AUC was
corrected also for the dose. That shows that rectal
suppository administration gives AUCs which are comparable
to the I.V. route. In other words, the absorption of

TABLE 3. TEST OF MANN-WHITNEY. VALUES OF PROBABILITY.

DOSAGE FORM COMPARED (AUC/D)	PROBABILITY (P)	DIFFERENCE STATISTICALLY SIGNIFICANT
I.V. SOLUTION 500 MG. RECTAL SUPPOSITORY 500 MG.	$p > 0.5$	NO
I.V. SOLUTION 500 MG. RECTAL SUPPOSITORY 750 MG.	$p = 0.036 < 0.05$	YES
RECTAL SUPPOSITORY 500 MG. RECTAL SUPPOSITORY 750 MG.	$p = 0.036 < 0.05$	YES

Metronidazole from the rectal suppositories is optimal.
These finding is in agreement with the results of Ioannides
(1981).

It is interesting to remark that all cases of 750mg
are in the **absorption** phase during all time studied while the
500 mg cases are not.

If we consider that the **elimination**   of
Metronidazole does not appear to be dose-dependent (Welling
and Monro, 1972 ; Wood and Monro, 1975), it seems that the
rate of absorption is lower for 750 mg dose. This point
needs to be confirmed by further studies.

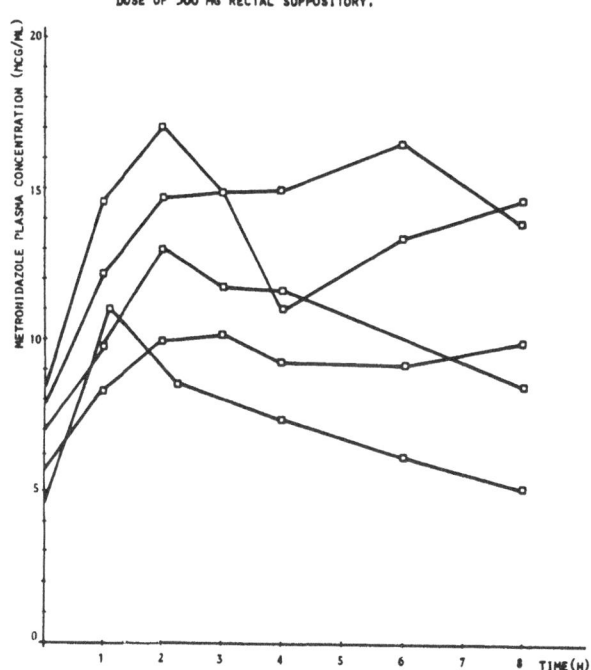

FIGURE 2. PLASMA CONCENTRATIONS OF METRONIDAZOLE AFTER THE SECOND
DOSE OF 500 MG RECTAL SUPPOSITORY.

The results of Table 4 brings the conclusion that at the operation time (6 hours before the second dose) there is no certainty that plasma concentration reachs levels higher than MIC (6.2 mcg ml). Consequently we are planning a new protocol for surgical prophylaxis to assure an effective plasma level. A new study is now in project to support this point.

TABLE 4. PLASMA CONCENTRATIONS OF METRONIDAZOLE ABOVE THE MIC (6.2 MCG/ML): PERCENTAGE OF TIME.

DOSAGE FORM	DOSE (MG)	PERCENTAGE
INTRAVENOUS SOLUTION	500	99.38
RECTAL SUPPOSITORIES	500	93.75
	750	100.00
RECTAL ENEMAS	500	74.44
	750	100.00

CONCLUSIONS

1.- According with this study there are no differences in terms of plasma concentration between i.v. solution 500 mg and rectal suppository 500 mg of Metronidazole.

2.- It seems that rectal suppository of 750 mg has slower absorption rate and bigger AUC than suppository of 500 mg. It seems also advisable to use this dosage form as loading dose in prophylaxis.

3.- In our Hospital i.v. Metronidazole costs 12,000 U.S. dollars per year, changing to rectal suppositories the cost will be of 150 U.S. dollars per year.

REFERENCES

Foster,G.E.; Bourke,J.B.; Bolwel,J. et al.(1981). Clinical and economic consequences of wound sepsis after appendicectomy and their modification by metronidazole or povidone iodine. Lancet, 1:769-71.

Goulton,J.; Baker,P.G. (1978). Multicentre study of Flagyl suppositories in the prevention of postoperative anaerobic infection. J. Int. Med. Res., 6: 471-5.

Ioannides,L.; Somogyi,A.; Spicer,J. et al.(1981). Rectal administration of Metronidazole provides therapeutic plasma levels in postoperative patients. New Engl. J. Med., 305: 1569-70.

Kabela,P.; Javensivu,P. et al.(1981). Comparative pharmacokinetics of oral and rectal dosage forms of metronidazole in man. Proceedings of the First European Congress of Biopharmacy and Pharmacokinetics, Clem, Ferrand,part 1: 416-9.

Marques,R.A.; Stanfford,B. et al. (1978). Determination of metronidazole and misonidazole and their metabolites in plasma and urine by high--performance liquid chromatography. J. Chromatogr. 146: 163-6.

Siegel,S. (1956). Non parametric statistics for behavioral sciences. Mc Graw-Hill, N.Y.

Stranz,M.H.; Bradley, W.E. (1981). Metronidazole (Flagyl IV^r
  Searle). Drug.Intell. Clin. Pharm., 15: 838-46.
Welling, P.G. & Monro, A.M. (1972). The pharmacokinetics of
  metronidazole and tinidazole in man. Arzneimittel
  Forschung, 22: 2129.
Wood, B.A. & Monro, A.M. (1975). Pharmacokinetics of tinida-
  zole and metronidazole in women after single oral
  doses. Br. J. Vener. Dis. 51:51.

Individual Factors influencing Aminoglycoside
Serum Levels

D.M. Devos[*], M. Lesne, M. Reynaert
University of Louvain, Brussels, Belgium

The purpose of this study was to determine the
factors influencing aminoglycoside serum levels
(Zaske, 1982). Different categories of patients
were considered. Serum levels were monitored as
mentionned before (Devos, 1982). Patients with
weight differing markedly from the ideal body
weight : obese patients have small volumes of
distribution (Vd), lean patients have large Vd.
Patients on parenteral nutrition and cancer patients
have Vd based on their actual body weight (ABW)
different from the usual Vd. Patients with third-
spacing often need a higher dose than that calculated on the basis of their ABW because of their
greater Vd : patients with edema, ascites, peritonitis, pneumonia,... Post- partum patients have
variable half-lives because of fluctuations in their
renal perfusion rates. Burn patients with normal
serum creatinine tend to have shorter half-lives.
Patients on hemodialysis : after an initial loading
dose, blood levels are drawn at 1, 6, 12 h and every 12 h thereafter until dialysis. A pre- and a
post-dialysis levels are collected as well as three
carefully timed levels during the hemodialysis
period. After dialysis a maintenance dose is
infused and a 1 h post-infusion level is drawn.
The elimination rates during and in between dialyses
are calculated. A dosage regimen is established
based upon the duration and the frequency of hemodialysis to maintain serum concentrations in an
acceptable therapeutic range. Predialysis and
1 h post-infusion levels are monitored regularly.
The dosage regimen is adjusted when necessary.

As the aminoglycosides pharmacokinetics is widely
variable, a close monitoring of serum levels can
help optimize the therapy. For the treatment of
patients undergoing intermittent HD, pharmacokinetic
data obtained during and between dialyses are of
great help to individualize the therapy and thereby
optimize patient care while minimizing toxicity.

[*] Research Assistant of the N.F.S.R.(Belgium)

References

1. Zaske D.E., Cipolle R.J. et al.
   Gentamicin pharmacokinetics in 1,640 patients.
   Antimicr.Ag.Chemother.,21, 407-411 (1982).

2. Devos D.M., Lesne M. et al.
   Aminoglycoside serum levels monitoring.
   Controversial Aspects in Aminoglycoside Therapy
   of Severe Infections. Brussels
   Abstract. In press (1982)

MONITORING THEOPHYLLINE PLASMA LEVELS

M.E. ARAÚJO PEREIRA

M.L. LOPES

H. FERREIRA
Serviços Farmacêuticos - Hospital de Santa Maria
1292 LISBOA CODEX - PORTUGAL

An asthmatic, 60 kg female patient had been receiving for several months 450 mg of aminophylline retard (Filotempo in Portugal), every 12 hours. Theophylline concentrations were measured in plasma samples according to an established protocol by EMIT (Syva). We obtained the following values : $C_{0-12}^{min.} = 12.2 \mu gml^{-1}$, $C_{0-12}^{max.} = 20.4 \mu gml^{-1}$, $K_{\overline{x}} = 0.061$, t 1/2 = = 10.3 h. Using 'the average concentration' equation, we concluded that for a desirable $C_{0-12}^{av} = 10 \mu gml^{-1}$ the schedule should be 400 mg of aminophylline every 12 hours, so, there was no need for correction of her dosage regimen. Later on, she tried another aminophylline "retard" (Euphyllin) receiving 350 mg every 12 hours. As we expected her theophylline levels were lower and she became more symptomatic.

ARAÚJO PEREIRA et al. :MONITORING THEOPHYLLINE PLASMA LEVELS

　　　　An asthmatic woman, thirty years old, weighing 60 kg,received
for several months 450 mg aminophylline "retard" (Filotempo in Portugal),
every twelve hours. She came to our out-patient service in order that
her theophylline plasma levels might be monitored.

　　　　In fact, we have an established protocol for "steady state"
which basically consists of getting blood samples every two hours, one
immediately before the first dose of the day and the others during the
interval between the two doses. Then theophylline concentrations were
measured by EMIT (Syva) (Table 1)

Table 1

TIMING OF SAMPLE COLLECTION (HOURS)	THEOPHYLLINE SERUM LEVELS μgml^{-1}
0	12.2
2	20.4
4	20
6	17.7
8	16.5
10	13.4
12	12.2

Figure 1 represents a semilogarithmic plot of the resulting data.

Figure 1 - Curve concentration time of Filotempo

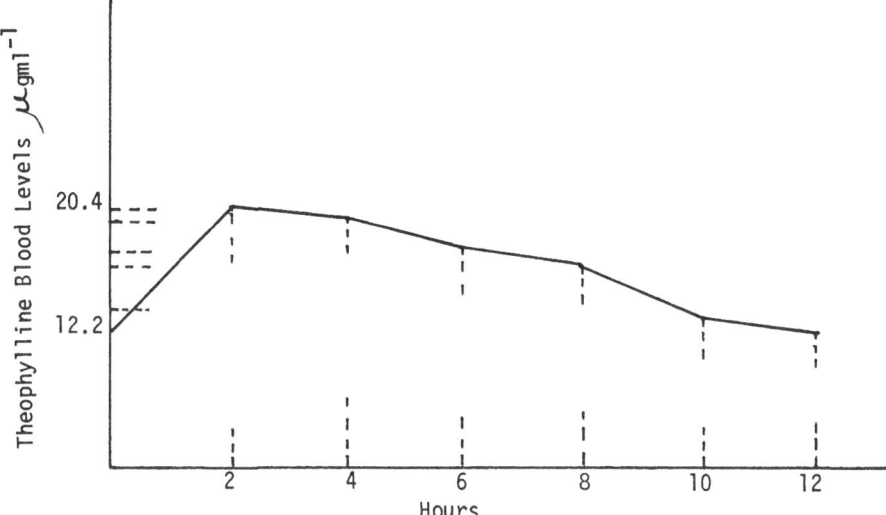

The area under the curve (AUC$_{0-12}$) was calculated using the trapeze rule, and its value is 200.4 mghl^{-1}. Clearance (Cl) was readily estimated using the following equation :

$$Cl = \frac{D}{AUC_{0-12}} \quad (1) \quad Cl = \frac{405}{200.4} = 2.02 \ \text{lh}^{-1}$$

D is the dose expressed in Mg.

We used then the "average concentration" equation to obtain the dose that will correspond to an average blood concentration of theophylline of 15 gml^{-1} :

$$FD = Cl \times \mathcal{T} \times C_{av} \quad (2)$$
$$FD = 0.033 \times 12 \times 15 = 6.05 \ \text{mg kg}^{-1} \ (\text{Theophyll.})$$
$\mathcal{T}$ is the interval between doses (12 h.)

So, we arrived at a schedule of 403 mg aminophylline every twelve hours. This result meant that our patient had a correct dosage regimen. Later on, she decided by herself to try another aminophylline "retard" (Euphyllin) taking 350 mg every twelve hours. She became symptomatic and once again we monitored her theophylline blood levels. (See table 2).

The peak levels were lower than we expected, perhaps on account of the shorter bioavailability of Euphyllin (E) which has been mentioned in the literature. We tried to calculate Euphyllin bioavailability compared to Filotempo (F). For this purpose the AUC_{0-12} of Euphyllin was determined also by the trapeze rule (Fig. 2).

Its value was 120.2 mghl^{-1}.

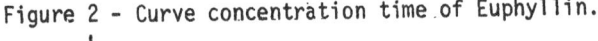

Figure 2 - Curve concentration time of Euphyllin.

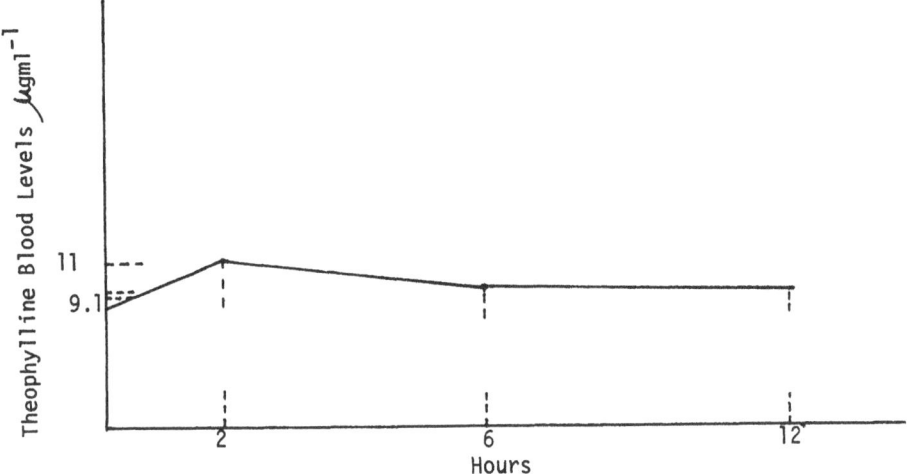

Table 2

TIMING OF SAMPLE COLLECTION (Hours)	THEOPHYLLINE BLOOD LEVELS μgml^{-1}
0	9.1
2	11
6	9.8
12	9.7

Then we used the following equation :

$$\frac{\text{Relative}}{\text{availability}} = \frac{\text{Area E}}{\text{Area F}} \times \frac{\text{Dose F}}{\text{Dose E}} \quad (5)$$

$$\frac{\text{R.a.}}{\text{of}}_{\text{Euphylline}} = \frac{120.2}{200.4} \times \frac{450}{350} = 0.77$$

This result achieved in a clinical case is in accordance with our expectations, but has not been statistically tested.

References

- Rowland, M.; Tozer, T.N. : Clinical Pharmacokinetics : concepts and application; Lea & Febiger, 1980, Philadelphia.

- Blaive, B. : Les theophyllines, Edition Marketing 1981.

- Wemhöner, S.; Oellerich, M.; Sybrecht, G.W. : Optimisation of theophylline therapy in obstructive respiratory disorders: Bio-availability and pharmacokinetics of various theophylline preparations - Han. Coll. of Medicine, West Germany.

COMPARISON OF FOUR PHARMACOKINETIC METHODS FOR
INDIVIDUALIZING PHENYTOIN DOSAGE

G.Zaccara, G.Arnetoli, G.Muscas, R.Zappoli
II Neurological Institute, University of Florence, Italy

A.Messori, G.Donati-Cori, E.Tendi
Hospital Pharmacy, USL 10/D, Florence, Italy

T.Valenza, C.Bartoli
Clinical Analysis Laboratory, USL 10/D, Florence, Italy

Abstract. During the past few years several pharmacokinetic procedures have been proposed for individualizing
phenytoin (PHT) dosage. Four of these are based on individualized estimation of PHT kinetic parameters in each patient
(1: "double reciprocal" method; 2: Ludden method; 3: "direct
linear plot" method; 4: Mullen & Foster method). We compared
accuracy of the above four methods in 23 epileptic patients
being treated with PHT. In order to compare the methods, for
each patient the Michaelis-Menten curve was fitted to the
experimental steady-state concentration-versus-dose data
points available; for each method the "goodness of fit" was
then evaluated by computation of the sum of the squared
residuals between fitted and experimental points (SSR). In
our patients, from the comparison of calculated SSR values,
the Mullen & Foster method proved to be capable of assuring
the best fit. Thus, on the basis of our data, this method
can be considered the most accurate one for individualizing
PHT dosage.

Since the 1970s, evidence has been provided that phenytoin
(PHT) has a dose-dependent pharmacokinetics which can be adequately
described by the use of the Michaelis-Menten model. While there is
agreement on the need to monitor PHT plasma levels, the use of an
appropriate kinetic procedure, which carries out individualized
calculation of kinetic parameters, is generally deemed to be necessary
as well due to the wide interindividual variations of PHT kinetic
parameters (namely the maximum rate of elimination, Vmax, and the
Michaelis-Menten constant, Km). Thus, during the last few years, several
pharmacokinetic techniques based on Michaelis-Menten principles have been
reported as a means of obtaining optimal individualized dosage more

easily. Four of these deserve particular consideration: the "double reciprocal" (DR) method, the Ludden (L) method (Ludden, 1976), the direct linear plot (DLP) method (Mullen, 1977), the Mullen & Foster (M&F) method (Mullen & Foster, 1979). Of all these techniques, the L method is the most widely accepted. In fact all the most recent clinical studies have adopted this technique (Ludden et al., 1977; Robinson et al., 1981; Bauer & Blouin, 1982).

To our knowledge, to date three papers have compared the clinical accuracy and reliability of the above methods for individualizing PHT therapy. The results are as follows: Murphy (1981) has found that L and DLP methods provide essentially similar results and can therefore be equally recommended; likewise Schumacher (1980) has shown that L, DLP, and M&F methods yield accurate and nearly identical predictions of Km and Vmax values (it should be noted that both these authors have compared other methods in their papers which, however, have generally proved less reliable than the above four methods). Conversely, Mullen and Foster (1979), based on simulated data, have shown the superiority of their proposed method. From this it appears that none of the above results has been found to be conclusive. Therefore the above data do not support a **clear** choice of a single method for use in routine clinical practice.

In order to establish which of the above four methods is the most accurate for clinical use, we applied and compared these methods in 23 epileptic patients treated with PHT alone or with PHT in association with other anticonvulsivants.

METHODS

For inclusion in our study the patient had to meet the following criteria: (i) the patient had been given at least three different PHT dosages with measurement of the corresponding steady-state concentration (Css); (ii) if drugs known to elicit variations in PHT Css were being administered concurrently, the dosage of these was not changed during the period of study; (iii) the patient was likely to be compliant with PHT dosage regimen.

For each patient, the Michaelis-Menten curve was fitted to the experimental data points by using either the DR, L, DLP, or M&F methods. For each method the "goodness of fit" was then evaluated by calculating the sum of squared residuals (SSR) between fitted and experimental points (each time the value of SSR was then divided by the number, n, of experimental data points available). Thus for each patient, the comparison between the methods was made on the basis of the parameter SSR/n calculated four times in accordance with the four methods. The calculation of the fitted values of Css has been developed by using some appropriate programmable calculator procedures (Ng, 1980; Valenza, 1982). In the case of the DLP technique, subjective bias in the graphic determination of parameters was eliminated by the use of a programmable calculator procedure carrying out the DLP interpolation on a mathematical, rather than on a graphical, basis.

RESULTS

Twenty-three patients were included in our study. The average number of Css-versus-dose data points per patient was 3.78.

In our patients, from the comparison of calculated SSR/n values, the M&F method proved to be capable of assuring the best fit. The statistical analysis (Rosenthal and Ferguson procedure) yielded the following results: the M&F method is significantly superior to both the DR (P=0.047) and L (P=0.032) methods. In comparison with the DLP method, the M&F method provided a lower average SSR/n value, though this difference is not significant (P=0.22).

No significant difference could be demonstrated in all the other pairwise comparisons between the methods.

DISCUSSION

Our data support the choice of the M&F method for use in

routine clinical practice, mainly because this method has given significantly superior results compared with both DR and L methods. Therefore our findings confirm the results obtained by Mullen and Foster with respect to simulated situations.

We believe that evidence may now support the choice of the M&F method for clinical use in individualization of PHT dosage. Probably the clinical advantages due to the use of a more accurate pharmacokinetic procedure are negligible in most cases. However, since most authors are currently employing the L method, which these and other data (Mullen & Foster, 1979) have demonstrated to be the least accurate, we feel that the use of a more reliable technique, such as the M&F one, may bring about some clinical benefits in the individualization of PHT therapy and that this technique should therefore be generally recommended.

REFERENCES

Bauer L.A. & Blouin R.A. (1982). Age and phenytoin kinetics in adult epileptics. Clin.Pharmacol.Ther.,31,301-4.
Ludden, T.M. et al. (1976). Optimum phenytoin dosage regimens. Lancet 1,307-8.
Ludden. T.M. et al. (1977). Individualization of phenytoin dosage regimens. Clin.Pharmacol.Ther.,23,228-32.
Mullen, P.W. (1977). Optimal phenytoin therapy: a new technique for individualizing dosage. Clin.Pharmacol.Ther.,23, 228-32.
Mullen, P.W. & Foster R.W. (1979). Comparative evaluation of six techniques for determining the Michaelis-Menten parameters relating phenytoin dose and steady-state serum concentrations. J.Pharm.Pharmacol.,31,100-4.
Murphy, J.E. et al. (1981). Clinical utility of six methods of predicting phenytoin doses and plasma concentrations. Am.J.Hosp.Pharm.,38,348-54.
Ng, P.K. (1980). Individualizing phenytoin dosage regimens using a programmable calculator. Am.J.Hosp.Pharm.,37,529-33.
Robinson, F.C. et al. (1981). Predicting individual phenytoin serum levels of patients seen in a private office practice. Neurology(Ny),31,761-3.
Schumacher, G.E. (1980). Using pharmacokinetics in drug therapy. VI: Comparing methods for dealing with nonlinear drugs like phenytoin. Am.J.Hosp.Pharm.,37,128-32.
Valenza, T. (1982). Program "Individualization of phenytoin dosage", Users' Program Library Europe, Hewlett-Packard, Geneva.

USE OF A CALCULATOR PROGRAM FOR INDIVIDUALIZED ESTIMATION
OF PHENYTOIN KINETIC PARAMETERS BY A LEAST-SQUARES TECHNIQUE

A.Messori, G.Donati-Cori, E.Tendi
Hospital Pharmacy, USL 10/D, Florence, Italy

G.Zaccara, G.Arnetoli, G.Muscas, R.Zappoli
II Neurological Institute, University of Florence, Italy

T.Valenza, C.Bartoli
Clinical Analysis Laboratory, USL 10/D, Florence, Italy

Abstract. In order to individualize phenytoin (PHT)
dosage in 24 epileptic patients, we applied a programmable
calculator procedure which is based on an iterative least-
squares technique for estimation of PHT kinetic parameters.
Our findings show that this programmable calculator procedure
allows optimal estimation of phenytoin kinetic parameters. In
comparison with the most used techniques for individualizing
PHT dosage (e.g. the Ludden method), the programmable
calculator procedure that we studied proved capable of
assuring an increased accuracy of calculated parameter
estimates. Since in several patients the calculator program
produced substantial improvement in the accuracy of
calculated parameter estimates, we believe that the use of
this calculator procedure should be recommended to all
physicians who have such a machine at their disposal.

Over the past decade many reports (Gerber & Wagner, 1972)
have shown that phenytoin (PHT) has dose-dependent pharmacokinetics
which can be adequately described by the Michaelis-Menten model.
Therefore, PHT has proved to be one of the few drugs for which the
assumptions of linear pharmacokinetics and applicability of the
superposition principle are not valid.

Individualization of PHT dosage thus involves some additional
difficulties when compared with the usual techniques for determining
individualized dosage regimens. Moreover, the well-demonstrated
interpatient variability of the Michaelis-Menten kinetic parameters of
PHT (namely the maximum rate of elimination, Vmax, and the Michaelis-
Menten constant, Km) further complicates the problem. For the above
reasons, for each patient individualized determination of Km and Vmax,

based on the measured PHT plasma levels, becomes a necessary step for the attainment of a proper PHT dosage regimen.

In order to determine for each patient a dosage capable of producing PHT plasma concentrations within the therapeutic range (approximately 10 to 20 mg/L), several pharmacokinetic techniques have recently been proposed, most of which are based on linear transformations of the Michaelis-Menten equation (Ludden et al., 1976; Mullen, 1977; Mullen & Foster, 1979; Robinson et al., 1982). The need to resort to a linear transformation derives from the fact that linearization converts the problem of parameter estimation from a non-linear regression analysis problem to a linear regression analysis one. But, unfortunately, the transformation descreases the accuracy of calculated parameter estimates.

However, a recent report (Messori et al., in press) has shown that the use of a suitable programmable hand-held calculator procedure allows for model parameter estimation according to a non-linear regression analysis based on an iterative least-squares technique. Since this iterative least-squares (ILS) method is not still available in print, a brief description is given here. The ILS method is based on the Gauss-Newton algorithm as modified by Hartley (1961). Therefore, on the one hand this method adopts the same theoretical approach as in computer programs such as NONLIN (Metzler et al., 1974); on the other, the use of a hand-held programmable calculator makes the ILS method easy to use in the clinical setting (the ILS method can be programmed onto a Hewlett-Packard 41 CV calculator or a Texas Instruments 59 calculator).

Since there is general agreement that iterative least-squares techniques are the most accurate method for model parameter estimation in all pharmacokinetic fitting procedures, we believe that the ILS method may find a role in the individualization of PHT dosage in routine clinical practice. The present article reports the results relative to clinical application of the ILS method in 24 patients treated with PHT.

METHODS

Although we examined for inclusion in our study all epileptic

patients treated with PHT at the II Neurological Institute of Florence,
only those patients who met the following criteria were in fact included:
-(a) the patient had to have received at least three different PHT
dosages with measurement of the corresponding steady state concentration (Css); PHT plasma concentrations were assumed to express
steady-state levels only when at least three weeks had elapsed since
initiation of therapy or dosage change.
-(b) if drugs known to elicit variations in PHT kinetics were being
administered concurrently, the dosage of these was not changed during the
period of study;
-(c) the patient was likely to be compliant with the PHT dosage.

PHT plasma concentrations were measured by a gas-
chromatographic technique.

Accuracy and reliability of the ILS method were assessed as
follows: for each patient, the Michaelis-Menten curve was fitted to the
experimental data points by using the ILS method; the "goodness of fit"
was then evaluated by calculating the sum of squared residuals (SSR)
between fitted and experimental points; each time the value of SSR was
then divided by the number, n, of the experimental data points available.

For comparison purposes, the value of SSR/n has been
calculated, in each patient, also on the basis of the Ludden (L) method,
which is the most commonly-used technique for individualizing PHT dosage.
Thus, for each patient, comparison between the L and ILS methods could be
made based on the parameter SSR/n calculated twice in accordance with the
two methods.

RESULTS

In comparison with the L method, the ILS method proved
capable of improving the fit in all 24 patients. In each case the ILS
method found the "true" sums-of-squares minimum, thus allowing obtainment
of the best parameter estimates. As compared to the L method, the ILS
method produced a mean per cent reduction of the value of SSR/n equal to

48.1 per cent.

For each patient, the square root of the SSR/n produced by the ILS method was calculated as well. As a result, this parameter was less than 1 mg/L in 19 cases (79 per cent) and between 1 and 2 mg/L in the remaining 5 cases (21 per cent).

The average number of Css-versus-dose data points per patient was 3.75.

DISCUSSION

Our findings demonstrate that the ILS method can be easily applied in routine clinical practice. As compared to the programmable calculator procedures previously described (Ng, 1980; King & Kaul, 1980), the ILS method on the one hand has demonstrated an equal ease of use; on the other, in many cases it has proved capable of providing parameter estimates which are considerably more accurate. The sole disadvantage is that the running time is relatively longer; however, in our patients it never exceeded 5 minutes.

In conclusion, we believe that, if the physician has a programmable hand-held calculator at his disposal, the ILS method may represent a valuable aid for individualization of PHT dosage; in fact, no practical difficulty derives from the sophisticated theoretical approach adopted by this method.

REFERENCES

Gerber, N. & Wagner, J.(1972). Explanation of dose-dependent decline of diphenylhydantoin plasma levels by fitting to the integrated form of the Michaelis-Menten equation. Res.Commun.Chem. Pathol.Pharmacol.,3,455-6.

Hartley, H.O. (1961). The modified Gauss-Newton method for the fitting of non-linear regression functions by least squares. Technometrics, 3,3:269-80.

King, W. & Kaul, A.F. (1980). Determining phenytoin dosage with the use of a programmable calculator. Drug.Intell.Clin.Pharm., 14,686-93.

Ludden, T.M. et al. (1976). Optimum phenytoin dosage regimens. Lancet 1,307-8.

Messori, A. et al. (in press). A new programmable calculator proce-
        dure for individualizing phenytoin dosage.
        Drug Intell.Clin.Pharm.
Metzler, C.M. et al. (1974). A package of computer programs for
        pharmacokinetic modeling. Biometrics,1974;30:562-3.
Mullen, P.W. (1977). Optimal phenytoin therapy: a new technique for
        individualizing dosage. Clin.Pharmacol.Ther.,$\underline{23}$,
        228-32.
Mullen, P.W. & Foster R.W. (1979). Comparative evaluation of six
        techniques for determining the Michaelis-Menten parameters
        relating phenytoin dose and steady-state serum
        concentrations. J.Pharm.Pharmacol.,$\underline{31}$,100-4.
Ng, P.K. (1980). Individualizing phenytoin dosage regimens using a
        programmable calculator. Am.J.Hosp.Pharm.,$\underline{37}$,529-33.
Robinson, F.C. et al. (1982). A graphic method for predicting individual
        phenytoin levels in an office practice. Ther.Drug.Monit.,
        $\underline{4}$,225-228.

ON THE IMPORTANCE OF REGULAR SERUM Al DETERMINATIONS IN
PATIENTS ON REGULAR HEMODIALYSIS (RHD).

J. Smeyers-Verbeke, D.L. Massart
Farmaceutisch Instituut, Vrije Universiteit Brussel (V.U.B.)

D. Verbeelen, J. Sennesael
Dienst Nefrologie, Academisch Ziekenhuis, V.U.B.

INTRODUCTION

During the last 10 years, increasing evidence has been given
that Al may be a toxic agent in patients with chronic renal failure
treated with regular hemodialysis. The increased interest wich has been
paid to Al has two causes :
- clinical disorders in patients with renal disfunction namely the dialysis encephalopathy and the osteomalacic bone disease, have been associated with an increased aluminium concentration in the organism.
- more sensitive and accurate techniques are becoming available for the
  determination of aluminium levels in biological samples.

Two potential sources of Al in patients on hemodialysis have
been proposed :
The water used to prepare the dialysis fluid (Flendrig et al. 1976)
Al can occur as a natural constituent in water or it can be added by the
water authorities as part of the water treatment process. Significant
amounts of Al can be transfered to plasma during dialysis since Al is
bound to a non-dialysable plasma component. This binding also precludes
the removal of Al from the patients during dialysis. To reduce Al to an
acceptable level reverse osmosis is the most effective method of removing
Al from the water. Therefore most dialysis centers are now using reverse
osmosis to avoid water borne toxicity especially from Al. It seems likely
that to minimize Al accumulation the concentration in the dialysis fluid
should not exceed 20 µg/l.
Gastrointestinal absorption of Al from aluminium containing phosphate
binders (Berlyne et al. 1970 ; Kaehny et al. 1977). They are widely
used in patients with renal disease to control plasma phosphate. It is
recognized that Al is absorbed from these compounds. In addition dialysis
encephalopathy and aluminium associated osteomalacia have been described
in non-dialyzed uremic patients who are taking phosphate binding agents.

Chronic Al loading, either from the use of contaminated water or from oral phosphate binders, contributes to an accumulation of Al in the body. Patients with renal failure have lost the capacity to excrete Al in the urine. Moreover hemodialysis is not an effective way for the removal of Al. As a result Al is transfered from the plasma to other tissue stores such as brain, bone, liver and muscle which may result in toxicity.

Therefore in order to reduce the risk of developing Al related toxicity it is important to minimize the exposure to Al. Regular serum Al determinations allow to estimate an overall exposure and when necessary, to take the apprpriate measures to reduce this exposure. We report the results of serum Al monitoring in our patients on RHD.

RESULTS AND DISCUSSION

In 1978 when we started with Al determinations in our patients on regular hemodialysis, high serum Al values where observed. Analyses were performed using an earlier described method (Smeyers-Verbeke et al. 1980). Aluminium in serum ranged from 38 to 682 µg/l. Seven of the patients had Al levels which exceeded 100 µg/l. At that moment one patient with a serum Al of 682 µg/l developed a dialysis encephalopathy with characteristic EEG abnormalities.

Since the water used for the preparation of the dialysis fluid contained less than 15 µg Al/l, the aluminiumhydroxide prescribed to all patients as phosphate binder, was thought to be responsible for the high serum Al concentrations in our patients. The effect of a reduction of the $Al(OH)_3$ prescribed is shown in figure 1.

Serum Al in all patients decreased. As a result serum phosphate increased but no patient developed however worsening of bone disease. Moreover an important decrease of the transfusion requirements in our patients was observed (Van Ingelgem et al. 1982). In all but one patient Al concentration decreased to below 100 µg/l. We believe that in order to reduce the risk of Al related clinical toxicity the serum Al concentration should be maintained below 100 µg/l since the three patients who had higher levels developed encephalopathy.

Patient 1 is a 55 year old male suffering from analgesic nephropathy. He was treated with RHD from 1976 to 1977 and from 1978 until his death in 1980. He took $Al(OH)_3$ to control serum phosphate. A routine serum Al determination showed a value of more than 600 µg/l. The patient was

warned against possible Al toxicity and was asked to reduce Al(OH)$_3$ which
he refused (the patient was a doctor himself). During a hospital stay an
EEG was performed and showed important disturbances. Three months later
the patient developed speech disorders and epilepsy. His condition de-
teriorated rapidly six months after the diagnosis of hyperaluminaemia was
established ; he died after neurological complications.

Patient 2 is a 32 year old male suffering from chronic glomerulonephritis.
He is treated with regular hemodialysis since August 1980. Medication
consist of Al(OH)$_3$ (50 ml/day) and hypotensives. One year after starting hemodialysis his family notices a strange behaviour and he also presents uncontrolled movement of arms and legs during dialysis. An EEG is
diffusely disturbed as in a metabolic disease. Serum Al is 210 µg/l at
that moment. Oral Al(OH)$_3$ administration is stopped and serum Al rapidly
drops to 5 µg/l one month later. At the same time the patients behaviour
returns to normal. In September he presents with a fracture of the pelvis
after falling from his bicycle. A bone biopsy taken at that moment shows
osteomalacia. Treatment with desferioxamine reverses this situation.

Figure 1

Serum Al monitoring in patients on RHD.
Effect of the reduction of Al(OH)$_3$ prescribed.

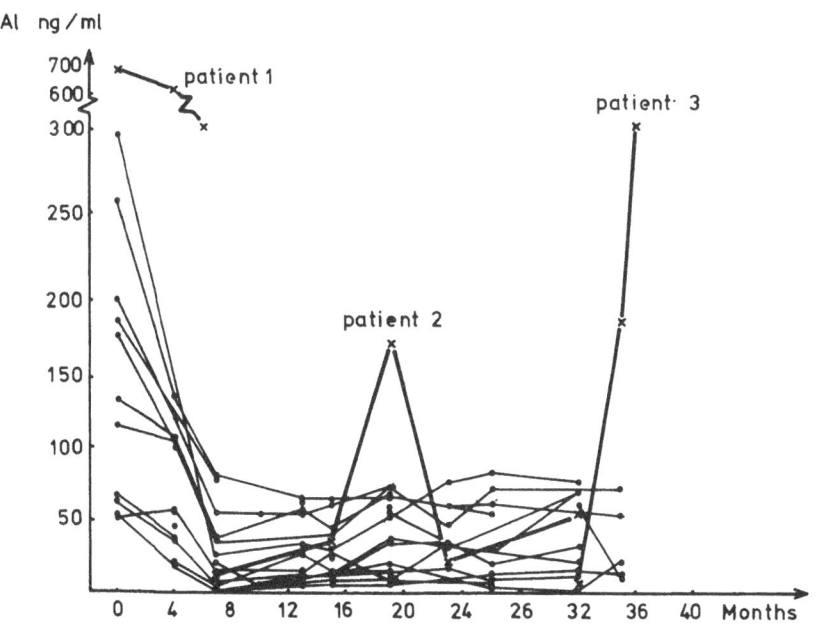

Patient 3 is a young woman of 36 years old. Chronic renal failure due to analgesic nephropathy was diagnosed in 1980. Because of terminal renal failure, regular hemodialysis treatment was started in May 1982. In July 1982, two months after starting RHD, aluminiumhydroxyde was prescribed because of hyperphosphataemia. Aluminium monitoring showed a tremendous increase of serum Al from 9 µg/l up to 409 µg/l. Meanwhile serum calcium increased markedly. Decrease of Al(OH)$_3$ administration and desferioxamine treatment reversed this dramatic situation.

From the results the value of regular monitoring of plasma and dialysis fluid aluminium in tracing patients at risk is evident. Regular aluminium monitoring enables the introduction of treatment to prevent further exposure and to reduce the risk of clinical toxicity. By this way we were able to detect 3 patients in whom serum Al was unacceptably high. Two of them were in a early stage of Al intoxication and appropriate treatment showed a reversal of the syndrome.

REFERENCES

Berlyne G.M., Pest D., Ben-Ari J., Weinberger J., Stern M. et al. (1970). Hyperaluminaemia from amuminium resins in renal failure. Lancet 2, 494-96.

Flendrig J.A., Kruïs H., Das H.A. (1976). Aluminium intoxication : the cause of dialysis dementia? Proc. Eur. Dial. Transplant Ass. 13, 355-61.

Kaehny W.D., Hegg A.P., Alfrey A.C. (1977). Gastrointestinal absorption of aluminium from aluminium-containing antacids. N. Engl. J. Ned. 296, 1389-90.

Smeyers-Verbeke J., Verbeelen D., Massart D.L. (1980). The determination of aluminium in biological fluids by means of graphite furnace atomic absorption spectrometry. Clin. Chim. Acta 108, 67-73.

Van Ingelgem D., Verbeelen D., Smeyers-Verbeke J., Sennesael J. (1982). Improvement of anaemia after reduction of aluminiumhydroxyde intake in patients on regular hemodialysis (RHD). XI th Annual Conference of the European Dialysis and transplant. Nurse Association Madrid, September 1982.

MANUFACTURE OF DIALYSIS CONCENTRATE AT THE LEVEL OF A HOSPITAL

Professor Y. DE ROECK-HOLTZHAUER
Chief Pharmacist of the Hospitals of Nantes
Professor of Industrial Pharmacy and Cosmetology with the
technical help of R. JAMAIN, Hospital Assistant.

Since the first trials of kidney dialysis in a nursing home of Lyons in 1962, the number of dialysed patients at home or in a hospital has been increasing regularly. The figures of 1982 show that in France 7,545 patients were dialysed in a hospital and 1,697 at home. Note also a broadening of the types of patients since quite old people will come three times a week for 6 hours to undergo the physical cleansing of blood. They range from 3 to 80 years old people in the Centre Hospitalier Regional of Nantes.

The first beds for dialysis were set up in Nantes in 1968 and at that time we used tins of 10 to 50 litres, and soon after 200 litre plastic tanks. The latter were delivered by trucks, coming from a pharmaceutic laboratory situated the other side of France.

Quite soon we had to face safety problems, as well at the analytical level as at the microbiological level. Moreover the tanks had been installed right in the middle of the psychiatric department and I remember I had to ask to circle the storage area with wire netting and to figure out a device to seal the upper openings of the tanks. There was no analytical checking when tanks arrived inasfar as they were guaranteed by an industrial pharmacist, although it was not a medicine submitted to market regulation but a preparation of a formula. No checking either after 15 to 20 days of storage in bad weather. No microbiological checking, but, now and then a sampling of the water used for dilution that was coming from a resin purifying apparatus. Quite often with a rate of contamination that necessitated immediate decontamination.

When the new service of dialysis was conceived in 1977-78, I was Chief Pharmacist of the Hospitals of Nantes and the man in charge of the Centre told me his projects and needs : a 21 bed ward, 17 of which were for chronic kidney deficient patients, and capable of treating 70 patients a week in turns, and 4 beds for occasonal patients, to cover a sanitary area of 750 000 inhabitants.

A quick calculation of needs led us to figure out the use of
2 000 to 3 000 litres of concentrate a week, with treatments that could
spread out in 3x8 hour periods each day.

Whence the first hypothesis of buying 200 litre tanks that could
be changed, that would be delivered by rail and then by road, with the problems of handling and failures of supplying that were entailed : holidays,
strikes... risks of contamination during the transportation, transfer car-
riage-truck, storage... We immediately decided to figure out the possibility
to manufacture the concentrate ourselves.

In the building of the Centre we proposed a manufacturing unit on
the ground-floor, together with mixing tanks, storage tanks, and a distribution and dilution circuit that was entirely automatic.

Moreover, two Electropur units provided us osmosed water in
quantities that were enough to clean the circuits and to manufacture the
concentrate, though we shall have to make a few comments later.

After the conception of the outline plan, am, we consulted suppliers and decided upon the following items :
I- a mixing funnel of 50 litres, with a Triblender diluter devised by GUERIN
II- a manufacturing tank in stainless steel of 2 000 litres, equiped with a
manhole, sterilized with steam, and using an axial mixer with a metallic
blade providing an horizontal brushing.
III- two groups of prefiltres of the Millipore type, with a porosity of
0,22 μ, necessary to secure a sterilizing sifting of the concentrate.
In spite of the work of BOWER and al. showing that such a highly salty concentrated aqueous solution could not be contaminated, we insisted on working
out a sterile manufacturing of the concentrate against the advice of the
Doctor that was in charge of the Centre and the hospital architect. Experience proved we were right.
IV- a first storage tank of 2 000 litres that should have been made of
stainless steel instead of polypropylene. We shall see that point later.
V- a second storage tank of 2 000 litres made of polypropylene to transfer
the controlled aqueous solution towards the service that used it.
VI- a storage tank of 3 000 litres made of polypropylene for storage of osmosed water within a closed circuit.
VII- a relay tank made of polypropylene to furnish the automatic diluter
with concentrate.
The estimated total cost of the plant was 200 000, and the real cost was
250 000 francs.
We are responsable only for the manufacturing proper, that is the stainless
tank and plastic tank n°I, in a manufacturing room that is close to where

raw materials are stored.

The chief of the medical service is responsible for the other tanks and the relay tank which are situated in the technical room of the dialysis service. We make sterility controls of these storage and dilution units on a continuous basis, of osmosed water and purified water, as well at the level of resistivity as from the point of view of the content in aluminium or microbial contamination. The tests for non-contamination are achieved by the warden of the hospital service up to the bed of the patient.

Let us recall the formula of the dialysis concentrate given in the 1976 edition of the Formulaire National Français :

Sodium chloride	409,500 kg	so the molar	Potassium	52,50
Potassium chloride	7,840	concentration is:	Sodium	47,25
Calcium chloride	26,840		Calcium	122,50
Magnesium chloride	10,640		Magnesium	52,50
Sodium acetate	333,200		Acetate	1225,00
Osmosed water, sufficient quantity			Chloride	3727,50

for 2 000 litres.

which secures a 1,5 meq/litre after dilution.

The high concentration of mineral salts was a problem for manufacturing and led us first to diluting salty elements at 60°centigrade, followed by sifting at the same temperature.

The content of a 82 H tank was suddenly troubled in the storage tank when it became cold and we had to throw it away. This led us to diluting and sifting at room temperature.

The manufacturing tank is automatically supplied with osmosed water during the night, thanks to a clock and a level valve. The device became necessary when the rhythm of manufacturing increased and we had to pump osmosed water outside the period between 7.00 and 10.00 p.m. when patients received their treatment.

The manufacturing tank in stainless steel must be cleaned regularly to take away the traces of rust and it must be passivated with a closed circuit of nitric acid at 10% for 60min. It is necessary then to enter the tank by the manhole in the upper part, in sterile clothes, using a rope ladder and a safety harness ; another assistant is compulsory outside the tank. A close and repeated cleansing uses about 3 000 litres of water which has been osmosed and sterilized. Samples of deposits of mud have been regularly taken from the bottom of the tank and analysed.

The polypropylene tanks are cleaned with a sponge used on the walls and the inside of the upper lid, with CO_3Na_2 or Pha-Labor at 5% after plunging in Javel water at 5%. A direct fogging of Buraton and Quatergenyl is made with no human intervention thanks to the appropriate apparatus. We had to make certain improvements as we noticed fungi contamination on the inside of the upper lid though the dialysis concentrate was not polluted. That is why the air openings in the upper part, which are necessary to transfer liquids from one tank to another, have been provided with a sterilizing filter of 0,5 µ. Nevertheless we note a systematic salty deposit on the inside of the lid, that we have to brush away. We think this is due to polypropylene itself which cracks and become porous little by little, even if it is invisible. We advise therefore other conceptors to insist on using stainless steel for storage and manufacturing tanks as well.

The decontamination of the various tanks, including the one used for dilution is made by turns every 5 weeks. It is undertaken during weekends because of the high quantity of water which is necessary for rinsing.

Let us point out the fact that we asked for an independant device providing distilled water that we can use at any time. Plugging on an osmoser of an insufficient capacity has proved an ill-purposed saving which causes our assistants to work at night or during the week-end.

Before and after the decontamination of tanks, we take samples on the surface with Rodac boxes for a microbiological analysis by contact. The results are filed in the following order.

The walls, the ceiling and the floor of the manufacturing rooms are decontaminated and surveyed by the same method of contact sampling. Trials had been made by sampling air on Oclogerm but we finally decided on the Rodac system. To stay in the C class, that is between 200 and 500 bacteria per m^3, it is necessary to decontaminate the air once a month.

Any micro leak at the level of valves entails an abundant white efflorescence which is normal as the aqueous solution is saturated with mineral salts. We note a regular deposit of rust due to the electrodes at the bottom of the tank which is closely rinsed.

The osmosed water is systematically sampled every week and the control form is filled: limpidity, pH, trials - chlorides, sulfates, alkaline content, heavy metals, ammonia -, dosage -aluminium-, searching for microbial cultures, yeast, mould.

Surveying the content in aluminium in the water used for dialysis was made compulsory in 1976 by the Formulaire National, and in 1980 by an addendum to the Pharmacopée Française dated 27 february 1980. The same article stipulates that pipes and a fortiori tanks can be made of plastified PVC, of high or low density polyethylene, or of polystyrene whereas copper, zinc bronze or iron is prohibited. Tanks must be opaque to avoid algae ; manholes must be locked and bacterial filters fixed on air openings.

This article, published in the Journal Officiel dated Ist april 1980 asks for an aluminium content inferior to 30 µg/litre. Whereas european projects think of imposing a maximum content of 200 µg/litre in drinking water. As soon as 1976 aluminium was suspected in the etiology of myoclonic encephalopathies happening to certain dialysed patients and observed since 1972. Aluminium can be a consequence of the treatment of city water by alumina during floculation, of the anti-corrosion device of certain water networks, of warming electrodes equipped with aluminium elements.

The content is checked each week with an atomic absorption spectrophotometer, and went above the accepted level only once or twice, reaching 50 ug - 100 ug so that the tank did not have to be thrown away, following the advice of the medical doctor who judges that only a highly chronic content in aluminium could be dangerous.

At various moments, we detected a microbial or fungi contamination that was more or less abundant, which did nor impressed our doctors, but led us to decide to decontaminate immediately the tanks and pipes. Our position is that it is useless to prepare a sterile concentrate if it is diluted 35 times in non sterile water.

The analytical control of the concentrate is made at various steps after dilution and mixing in tank A, with a transfer in tank B,... in tank B before transfer in tank C.

A rate error of more or less 5% is legally tolerated. Some errors can reach 4,5%, particularly with calcium because of the hygrosgopic nature of these salts which is variable. The important weights cause us to group our buyings by 15 tons on months, with sacks of 50 kg whose content in water is not constant ; sacks can harden or liquefy. Few suppliers cater for our demands so that we have to buy from foreign countries through French circuits. We also have to point out the important problems of handling which needs pallets and fork lift trucks, since justone preparation necessitate 788 kg of mineral salts, that is 20 sacks of 50 kg that have to be emptied in the mixing funnel.

The constant increase of needs led us to prepare one tank a week that is, in spite of holidays, 50 tanks a year. The manufacturing started in decembre 1978, in 1979 33 tanks were prepared, 43 in 1980 and 1981 and 45 have been prepared today for 1982.

To increase even further the rhythm of treatment, the hospital doctor is thinking of modifying his plant so that he will not have on one pool of solution that he has to store, but on a dilution prepared extemporaneously for each apparatus. The effect would be, without increasing the number of people working at the hospital, to meet with an increased number of patients. And, above all, to make the system more flexible since an individualized complimentary supply, in the shape of tins, allows to modify the composition of the dialysate according to the patient.

As a summary : safer realisation

undoubtedly more profitable process ; cost of the operation 250 000 francs that are reimbursed in less than 2 years.

safety of the system...

Difficulties will arise at the level of the maintenance of the composition of the aqueous solution; severe precautions : sterilized water and instruments, 2 tanks out of 160 have been thrown away up to now, cleanliness of rooms, quality of the osmosed water and duration of the osmoser, content in aluminium of the water with accidental increases, constancy of the formula, which does not allow the person in charge of such a unit to change regularly the formula of the dialysate.

For instance, the chief of the service wanted a higher potassium content of 2 meq/l instead of 1,5 meq/l. We did not prepare it because of the already highly saturated of the solution and the risks of precipitates that had already been observed during the preliminary trials in the laboratory.

As a conclusion, the realisation shows the excellent collaboration between an hospital doctor and an hospital pharmacist and his technical staff to meet with the demand of therapeutics. Only a pharmacist, aware of his responsibilities and working with a highly qualified staff can achieve such a manufacturing.

REFERENCES

AAMI KIDNEY STANDARDS SUBCOMMITTEE,
Revised standards for hemodialysis, Ass.A.I.O., 1974, 20 B,
770-3.

BECKER A. , DELION F. ,LEBAS M. ,
Pharmaceutic aspects of the incidence of various treatments of
purifying water on the quality of water used in hemodialysis,
Magazine of the ADSHSO, 1982, 7, n°1, 71-8.

BOWER et coll.,
Bactericidal properties of the concentrated artificial kidney
bath solutions,
Applied Microbiol., 1976, 14, n°1, 45-8.

EAU,   Oct. 1976 Formulaire National, Add. 30 to the Pharmacopea
J.O. 1-04-80.

HAAS T., MEYRAND B., DONGRADI B.,
A comparative study of in vivo performances of 15 hollow fibre
dialysers,
RBM, 1981, 3, n°1, 39-41.

HARTMANN P.,How to figure out a plant for the treatment of water used in
kidney dialysis,
Techn. Hosp., 1979, 410, 37-41.

JUNGERS P., ZINGRAFF J., MAN N.K., DRICKE T.,
Essentials on hemodialysis, Paris, Maloine, 1978.

LACOMBE,   Blood pumps used in hemodialysis,
RBM 1981, 3, n°6, 423-25.

LEBAS J., The controls of waters in a hospital,
Pharmacie Hosp., 1982, n°186, 97-100, n°187, 65-8.

MAISON C., Analysed osmosed water : 100 microorganisms/ml, tolerated limit
Kidney Standards Subcommittee.

MERY D., POUILLOT M.J., MAISON C.,
The problems of the microbiological surveying of liquids used
in dialysis,
Pharmacie Hosp., 19870, n°61, 15-20.

HOSPITAL PREPARATION OF INJECTABLE DRUGS BY MEANS OF A MULTI-ADDITIVE PUMP

J. WODELET
PHARMACIST
ERASME UNIVERSITY HOSPITAL
BRUSSELS BELGIUM

" OBJECTIVE "

TO PREVENT THE RISK OF ACCUMULATION OF THE DRUG IN THE BODY WHEN MULTIPLES DOSES OF FENTANYL[R] ARE INJECTED DURING THE COURSE OF LONG LASTING SURGICAL PROCEDURES. (RESPIRATORY DEPRESSION), THIS MULTIPLE INJECTIONS HAS BEEN REPLACED BY CONTINUOUS INTRAVENOUS INFUSION OF FENTANYL[R].

WE MAKE A PHARMACEUTICAL PREPARATION OF CONTINUOUS INTRAVENOUS INFUSIONS FROM FENTANYL[R] AMPOULES AND A FILTRATION TO ELIMINATE GLASS PARTICLES

" METHODOLOGY "
- FABRICATION UNDER LAMINAR AIR FLOW.
- SURGICAL HANDS WASHING.
- CONNECTIONS
- PUMPING, STERILIZING FILTRATION AND FILLING OF PLASTIC CONTAINERS WITH A MULTI-ADDITIVE PUMP.

" RESULTS AND CONCLUSIONS "
- THE FILTRATION SHOWED GLASS PARTICLES ON THE FILTER MEMBRANE (SLIDE).
- FINALLY THE SOLUTION CAN BE ADMINISTRED WITHOUT RISKS TO THE PATIENT AND ALLOWS A " STRESS FREE " ANESTHESIA.
- THIS TECHNIQUE PROVIDES A READY-TO-USE SOLUTION WITHOUT GLASS PARTICLES (PARENTERAL ADMIXTURE SERVICES).

HOW TO DETECT PHYSICO-CHEMICAL INCOMPATIBILITIES
IN I.V. ADMIXTURES

D. Koechel
Apotheke Stadtkrankenhaus
Kanzlerstraße 2 - 6
7530 Pforzheim   West Germany

Abstract. Mixing parenteral solutions compatibility
can be attested only, when there are no losses in
physico-chemical stability, no mutual chemical
influences and no pharmacological interactions.
It will be therefore useful to examine physico-
chemical reactions, before testing a new parenteral
combination. As the value of compatibility studies
is also limited to the manner of measuring method,
the following standard programme should be used by
the clinical pharmacist. Immediately before and
after mixing, also 2, 6 and 24 hours after mixing
parenteral solutions, infusion solutions or infusion
and parenteral solutions must be studied in a
laboratory: pH-level, colour index, possible
precipitation, floculation or crystallisation,
Tyndall effect and measured values of spectrophotometer. The appraisal should be: "Not miscible,
miscible when consumed within 6 or 12 hours, mixture
without change during 24 hours". It is not intended
to give recommendations for mixing new parenteral
combinations with this appraisal. The hospital
pharmacist however should be able to give advice,
if admixtures should not be done.

Mixing parenteral solutions, infusion solutions or
parenteral and infusion solutions like amino acids, dextrose,
electrolytes, trace elements, vitamin supplements, lipids,
Insulin, Heparin or drugs as they are commonly used specially
in total parenteral nutrition, three important aspects should
be considered: Avoidance of bacterial contamination,
avoidance of particle invasion and maintenance of the
therapeutic effectiveness.

Whereas microbial contamination and particle
invasion can be prevented by the use of laminar-flow-boxes
and aseptic conditions, the therapeutic effectiveness of the
components in such solutions is maintained only, when there

are no losses in the physico-chemical stability of the
solution or emulsion system, no mutual chemical influences
and no pharmacological interactions.

This is the question of incompatibilities and
interactions.

Particular significance is due to the physico-
chemical stability, because physico-chemical miscibility
alone shows whether parenteral solutions should be mixed
or not at all. When a new combination is planned, whose
compatibility is not yet attested, it would be beneficial for
the hospital pharmacist to examine physico-chemical reactions.
These physico-chemical incompatibilities can be visible or
masked.

V i s i b l e physico-chemical incompatibilities
are mostly produced by admixtures of aqueous and oily
solutions, degradation of solubility by "salting out" effects,
degradation of solubility by pH-deviations, reactions of
active substances with solutes or floculation of emulsion
globules by changes in particle size distribution.

M a s k e d physico-chemical incompatibilities can
be produced by adsorption reactions, dissolution reactions,
hydrolysis, formation of complexes or not wanted reactions
with halogen and chemical transformation.

All possible reactions in parenteral combinations
must be considered as reaction of infusion bottle, transfusion
system, basic vehicle or solvents with a drug, reaction of a
drug or an adjuvant with components of the infusion fluid,
reaction of an infusion bottle or basic vehicle with a solvent
and reaction of several basic vehicles.

The examination of physico-chemical miscibility is
the one and only possibility to test a new combination before
starting the application, should information about physico-
chemical or pharmacological incompatibilities not be available.
If new combinations are considered, on recommendation of
Beisbarth (1977) the following standard programme should be
taken, because the value of compatibility studies is generally
limited due to the concentration of additives, the

environmental conditions, time and manner of the measuring
method.

First of all the environmental conditions and the
chosen concentration in the test must agree to the clinical
use. Also the infusion rate must be considered. Then in a
final volume of 100 ml the parenteral solution, infusion
solution or parenteral and infusion solution are mixed
together in a laboratory.

Immediately before and after mixing, also 2, 6 and
24 hours after mixing, pH-level, colour index, possible
precipitation, floculation or crystallisation, Tyndall effect
and measured value of spectrophotometer are checked.

The measure of pH-level is important, because each
drug needs for its stability and concentration a special
pH-range. Whereas in the closed vial will be an optimal
situation, depending on titratable acidity and buffer capacity
of the infusion fluid, after mixing perhaps another pH-value
can occur, where dissolution or other incompatibilities take
place. To show physico-chemical stability, pH-values should
not change more than two tenths, in buffered or extreme acid
solutions even not more than one tenth.

In interpretating the result, one should definitely
consider an interaction with the carbon dioxide in the air
which cannot be eliminated under the present test conditions.
The influence of carbon dioxide may be noticed in the test,
depending on the present solution system. However later in
clinical use, it will not usually have an effect.

To control the colour index it is better to make
use of the colour standard solutions of the European
Pharmacopeia. In our programme two further standards for pale
tints are added to the six assigned stages of the colour
intensity. Also one characterisation "W" like water-clear was
added to the different colour characterisations. More than
one grade of shade-change should set one thinking. It is
difficult to see little colour changes.

Whereas mixing 30 ml Theophyllin-Ethylenediamine in
500 ml 5 % Glucose solutions produces at once and after 8

hours no difference   in colour appearance, adding 30 ml
Theophyllin-Ethylenediamine (equivalent to three ampoules of
240 mg) to 500 ml 5 % Fructose solution shows after 8 hours
a slight yellow gleam. Only the colour standard proves
whether colour change took place or not. in our case the
colour changed more than two grades. This was not permissible.

Precipitation is often also not seen at once. The
next example shows you therefore the significance of time.
Mixing 40 ml Calcium Chloride 7,45 % (corresponding 40 mmol
Calcium ions in 1 litre) to a solution with 5 mmol Phosphate
ions in 1 litre, precipitation will first be noticed after
two hours.

Floculation or crystallisation are also frequently
not perceptible to the eye, when the process begins.
Therefore spectrophotometer measures should be made at
550 nm. This wave-length is comparable in its effectiveness
to the effect of the dispersion filter. It is advantageous
for nephelometric use. On the other hand Tyndall effect
provides the answer, if phase change should occur.

In order to safely document the measured values, it
would be practicable to use an index card. If known, masked
physico-chemical or pharmacological changes should have an
influence on the interpretation of the results. Supplements
can made on the index card too.

The hospital pharmacist must then make his decision
as to whether the mixture is physico-chemical compatible or
not. The final assessment must include the maximum assigned
time of infusion, time of preparation and handling and an
adequate time reserve.

The appraisal should be: "Not miscible, miscible
when consumed within 6 or 12 hours, and mixture without
change during 24 hours". Using this definition prevents from
misinterpreting the results. It is not intended to give
recommendations for mixing new parenteral combinations with
this appraisal. The hospital pharmacist should only give
advice if admixtures should not be done.

The results can be transferred onto tabular forms

and discussed by pharmacists and physicians. As usual the
physician should have the last decision if wanting to use
the combination.

Reference list.
Beisbarth, H. (1977). Kompendium für Infusionstherapie und
        bilanzierte Ernährung, 16, 73. Erlangen: Pfrimmer+Co
Beisbarth, H. & Köchel, D. (1979). Arzneizusätze zu
        Infusionslösungen und deren Kompatibilität.
        Infusions-Journal, 2, No. 3.
Köchel, D. (1980). Probleme bei Arzneigemischen.
        Wehr-Medizinische Monatsschrift, 24, No. 10, 319.
Köchel, D. (1981). Kompatibilität und Inkompatibilität von
        Arzneigemischen. Schleswig-Holstein. Ärzteblatt, 34,
        No. 7, 326 - 332.

PREPARATION OF AN ENEMA CONTAINING METAMINOSALICYLIC ACID

E. De Schouwer, J. Hoogmartens, M. Dooms, P. Bruyneel
Dept. of Pharmacy, University Hospital St Rafaël, Capucynenvoer, 3000 Louvain, Belgium

Metaminosalicylic acid (5-aminosalicylic acid, 5-ASA) was used already for several years, being the active metabolite of salicylazosulfapyridine (Salazopyrine^{TM}), a product used by the treatment of Crohn's desease and ulcerative colitis.

Recently rectal administration of 5-ASA has been described (1, 2). In the University Hospital of Louvain a double blind study is carried out with enemas containing 1,5 g/100 ml 5-ASA (*) compared with a placebo. Difficulties arose when imitating the brown colour of 5-ASA for the preparation of the placebo. However this colour was caused by impurities, which may be toxic. That's why we developed a method to purify 5-ASA, getting an almost white product, which was safer to use and much easier to imitate when compounding a placebo.

1. A.D.Azad Khan,J.Piris, S.C. Truelove.(1977)
   An experiment to determine the therapeutic moiety of
   sulphasalazine.
   Lancet,2,892.
2. M.Campieri,G.A.Lanfranchi,G. Bazzocchi, et. al.(1981)
   Treatment of ulcerative colitis with high dose
   5-aminosalicylic acid enemas.
   Lancet,2,270

(*) Obtained from Aldrich Europe,Beerse.